METABOLIC TOXEMIA
OF
LATE PREGNANCY

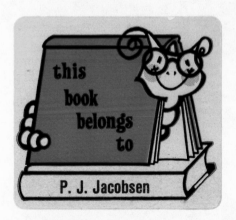

METABOLIC TOXEMIA
OF
LATE PREGNANCY

A Disease of Malnutrition

By

THOMAS H. BREWER, M.D.

Keats Publishing, Inc.   New Canaan, Connecticut

METABOLIC TOXEMIA OF LATE PREGNANCY
A Disease of Malnutrition

Copyright © 1982 by Thomas H. Brewer, M.D.

All Rights Reserved
ISBN: 0-87983-308-4
Library of Congress Catalog Card Number: 82-82321

Printed in the United States of America

Keats Publishing, Inc.
27 Pine Street
New Canaan, Connecticut 06840

CONTENTS

This book is respectfully dedicated to:

The obstetrical patients of Charity Hospital, New Orleans, Louisiana, to those of Jackson Memorial Hospital, Miami, Florida, and to those of the Richmond Health Center, Richmond, California, from whom I learned many basic facts about metabolic toxemia of late pregnancy;

James H. Ferguson, M.D., Professor and Chairman of the Department of Obstetrics-Gynecology, University of Miami School of Medicine, Jackson Memorial Hospital, Miami, Florida, who first taught me the classical ideas about this common disease of pregnancy when I was a medical student at Tulane University School of Medicine, New Orleans, and who later provided opportunities for my obstetrical training and clinical research studies of this problem at Jackson Memorial Hospital; and

To the memory of Claude Bernard, French physiologist, the real Father of Modern Scientific Medicine, who taught me through his classic writings about medical research to "look on the other side of the coin."

PREFACE TO THE FIRST EDITION

*The disease prevails among the underprivileged and
is seldom seen among well-fed and well-cared-for patients.*

WITH THESE words Mengert and Tweedie in 1964 introduced
their report on "acute vasospastic toxemia: therapeutic nihilism."
This generalization has been widely accepted by clinical obstetricians
in the United States, but little scientific effort has been expended to
answer the question: How is this so? Popular theories of the pathogenesis of this disease, "toxemia of pregnancy," have totally ignored its
obvious relationship to poverty, malnutrition, ignorance and socioeconomic deprivation. This work provides part of the scientific answer
to that question and will lay the foundation upon which more complete biochemical knowledge may be rapidly acquired.

This disease which is responsible for a number of maternal deaths
and even more fetal deaths in our nation each year is no longer a
complete "enigma." We have acquired enough scientific knowledge
to prevent it completely. I hope that this work will convey this knowledge to a significant number of physicians responsible for the care of
pregnant women. I also hope that this knowledge will be a stimulus
to public health and political authorities to take the steps necessary to
improve the maternal health of large numbers of American women
now living in poverty.

I want to express my deep appreciation to Mr. Payne Thomas for
his encouragement and for making possible the publication of this
work.

THOMAS H. BREWER

INTRODUCTION TO THIS NEW EDITION

Like many doctors with the M.D. degree, I was told in medical school and internship training that the unborn baby, like a parasite, would "steal" whatever it needed from the body of the host mother. "A tooth for a baby."

Now after thirty years of drug-oriented practice of pediatrics I have discovered—much of it from the research of Tom Brewer—that the pregnancy is really a launching pad for the infant. If the nine months has been inadequate in nutrition or has been too stressful, the infant suffers and will reveal this hurt with a seige of colic, a lifetime of allergies, frequent infections or inappropriate behavior. We drug all these children—sedatives, antihistaminics, antibiotics, psychotropics—because that is our training; we treat with medicines. But at the same time we should have been signaling the obstetricians to let them know that something was amiss. But we didn't have the insight nor the tools of research to indicate who or what was to blame.

"Some kids are sick a lot," we told the parents somewhat sheepishly. Now we ask, without trying to stir up any guilt, "Were you comfortable in the pregnancy?" or "How much did you gain?" or "Did you have nausea, vomiting, fevers, drugs, cramps or stress?" "How many months separate the pregnancies?" and most important, "What did you eat?"

Recently a mother told me when I was trying to find some valid reason for her child's severe, multiple allergies: "I'm not sure about stress when I was pregnant with him; I was 14 years old then." That's stress! Her *own* body wasn't even finished.

Stress and a poorly nourished pregnancy frequently lead to a sickly, allergic baby. Apparently the adrenal glands of the infant are depleted simultaneously with the depletion of the mother's adrenals. Her perception of stress is the important criterion.

One obvious stress is the metabolic toxemia that can be so easily avoided. This condition is a stress and will lead to further depletion of the woman's body. Stress leads to a disease and the disease leads to stress; a "Catch 22."

From my standpoint, if the mother survives the ravages of toxemia and the baby is still intact after this tumult, she is usually unable to nurse the poor thing because of her exhaustion. These are the very children who should be nursed for one to two years because they especially need this protection from allergies and infections.

We now have enough information to be able to throw some weight of responsibility back to the obstetricians, busy though they are with treating toxemia (usually preventable), abruptio placentae (probably nutrition based), premature labor (most of it could be avoided), and doing Caesarians (not all of them are necessary). We must get their attention. They have got to pay more than lip service to nutrition.

But for years Tom Brewer has been trying to get the attention of his OB peer group. They think him a maverick. "We have drugs; we don't need Tom."

My plan: find organizations and people who will underwrite a free gift of this book to every girl who is 13 years old or has had her first menstrual period. If these girls could just learn the value of a good diet—for their own bodies but also to assure that they will more likely have a healthy, happy child.

Our country will then be full of people free of sickness, aches, allergies and meanness. The obstetricians will get the credit, but Keats Publishing and Tom and I will know. And I promise I will send a nice letter to these generous donors saying: "You are OK. Have a good day. I love you."

Lendon Smith
Chicago, June 1982

FOREWORD TO THIS NEW EDITION

There is a great void in medical education today. I refer to specific training in the preventive aspects of nutrition. Several years ago I surveyed the curricula and course offerings of a random sample of 38 American medical schools. My findings confirmed fully the situation revealed by the Select Subcommittee Hearings of the United States Senate, January 30, 1979. In essence it isn't done. Many programs do not formalize preventive medicine in general. I found only one school with a good program directed at applied clinical nutrition.

Nonetheless, one sees growing evidence of awareness among American physicians on the importance of nutritional support in the *treatment of disease*. One good example is the salutary effect of specific nutritional support during cancer chemotherapy. Another is the relationship of nutritional status and survival following surgery for perforated duodenal ulcer.

If nutritional preparation for stressful events makes sense *en passant*, is it not at least equally logical to make that preparation in advance whenever possible?

The flaw in the plan is the easily demonstrated lack of a working knowledge of applied nutrition on the part of physicians generally. Even when a doctor has this skill, one has to deal with often deep seated cultural bias, lifelong (bad) habits, and for some, the cost of better foods, especially good quality protein.

Of even greater importance is the role of good nutrition in pregnancy. Human fetal growth and development are a majestic exercise in the accumulation of protein. Good animal husbandmen will not breed stock showing poor nutrition and will feed pregnant stock specially constructed diets. The same is true of breeders of animals for research, where uniformity of genetic, nutritional and physical attributes are required for the validation of experiment.

Human pregnancy nutrition is a subject in disarray, not for lack of certain basic information, but because it is so largely ignored in practice. The nutritional history of the obstetric patient may be taken by a trained associate, but nutritional instruction must come from the physician. In this activity the obstetrician reassesses the patient's command of the subject, and uses his or her authority role to reinforce the instruction.

Thomas H. Brewer, M.D., the author of this interesting and remarkable book, is one of a handful of pioneers of this educative approach. He stands in a long line of noted physicians making contributions to this field, such as Eva Dodge, John Ebbs, Winslow Tompkins, Reginald Hamlin, J. F. Kerr Grieve, James Henry Ferguson, Robert A. Ross, Maurice B. Strauss.

The work also commends itself to the practicing obstetrician because it shows what just one doctor can do to find evidence to support an insight derived from careful reflection on a clinical problem.

Dr. Brewer provides evidence that protein-calorie malnutrition is a causal factor of high significance in the so-called "mysterious disease," eclamptogenic toxemia, or gestosis. He points out the necessity of adequate salt intake to meet the physiological expansion of the extracellular water compartment of pregnancy. This awareness leads naturally to complete avoidance of saluretic diuretics, use of which reduces this compartment. In like fashion increased amounts of protein, iron and ascorbic and folic acid are required to build up expansion of the red cell mass which occurs, not to mention the fetal needs.

Equally flawed is the old concept of fetus as perfect parasite. If the mother does not receive adequate nutritional support from her environment, both mother and fetus will suffer the harmful consequences. The book that follows is an excellent point of departure for interested professionals in their quest for enhancing awareness on this vital subject.

Douglas R. Shanklin, M.D.
Formerly Professor Obstetrics and Gynecology,
University of Chicago and Pathologist-in-chief,
Chicago Lying-in Hospital
June, 1982

METABOLIC TOXEMIA
OF
LATE PREGNANCY

CHAPTER 1

INTRODUCTION

THIS BOOK will develop a scientific *point of view* about toxemia of late pregnancy. It will clarify and simplify the clinical problems associated with pregnancy hypertension, proteinuria and generalized edema, problems which commonly confront physicians actively engaged in the clinical practice of obstetrics. Thousands of medical articles have been published about this disease in the past twenty years, yet it has remained "the ancient enigma of obstetrics." Hundreds of articles are pouring forth each year on this subject from many nations. We are in need of a framework or basic foundation upon which we can evaluate these contributions, create an accurate picture of these problems and apply our most scientific knowledge in daily practice for the health and welfare of our patients. I think the material presented herein will be of direct practical use to clinical physicians and all persons concerned with the care of pregnant women; it should be of interest and value to persons working in the fields of public health and preventive medicine.

Claude Bernard wrote in 1865:

> Science should always explain obscurity and complexity by clearer and simpler ideas.

It is the purpose of this volume to point out the simple direct relationship between poor nutrition in pregnancy and the development of toxemia of late pregnancy. This can be done only by establishing a more precise, scientific conception of "toxemia of pregnancy" as a *disease entity,* with careful attention to its complex clinical differential diagnosis. Scientific evidence will be presented which clearly indicates that toxemia of late pregnancy is a disease of nutritional deficiency mediated through hepatic dysfunction and that the bacterial flora of the maternal gastrointestinal tract, as well as the steroid hormones (estrogens and progesterone) produced by the placenta, play a contributing role in its pathogenesis. The signs and symptoms of this disease will be viewed as the outward manifestations or *end results* of fundamental disturbances in metabolism, primarily in the metabolism of hepatic cells, brought on by malnutrition. Hence the disease is termed *Metabolic Toxemia of Late Pregnancy.*

The point of view presented here is the result of over ten years study of this disease process in over 500 women with "toxemia of pregnancy." A large percentage of these women lived in our southern states in the lowest socioeconomic class. I have found it necessary, as my own clinical experiences developed, to challenge many of the basic assumptions firmly established in clinical obstetrical thinking here in the United States, assumptions which I believe are actually blocking further creative research in elucidating the biochemical basis of this common complication of late pregnancy, false assumptions which often lead the clinician astray and prevent him from giving his patients the most scientific and effective care.

For many years the *signs* of this disease process have been used in an attempt to explain its pathogenesis; terms such as "acute vasospastic toxemia" indicate the great emphasis which has been placed by obstetrical authorities on the single clinical manifestation of *hypertension.* One of the most vexing of unproved assumptions about toxemia of pregnancy is the assumption that hypertension, or its physiologic counterpart, "vasoconstriction," *causes* "anoxia" or "hypoxia" in various tissues and organs and thus brings on tissue damage, convulsions and other manifestations of the disease. Any obstetrician with extensive clinical experience with severe metabolic toxemia of late pregnancy (henceforth abbreviated MTLP) has seen patients have toxemic convulsions with normal blood pressures or with borderline elevations. There is *no* scientific evidence that the endothelial lesions found in the liver, kidneys, adrenals, lungs, heart or brain of a woman dead of MTLP are *caused* by "hypoxia." There is no scientific evidence that "hypoxia" or a reduction in utero-placental blood *precedes* the onset of clinical toxemia.

Clinical and biochemical evidence will be presented to show conclusively that MTLP *cannot* be adequately explained by the currently popular theory of "utero-placental ischemia," nor by "uterine overdistension," nor by "increase in intrauterine pressure," nor by a "utero-renal reflex," nor by "placental infarcts," nor by "placental insufficiency," nor by "psychological stress," nor by (shades of the Dark Ages) "atmospheric, telluric conditions."

Certain common clinical assumptions about MTLP being a disease somehow *caused* by primiparity, obesity, multiple pregnancy, hydramnios, excess salt intake, chronic hypertension, chronic renal disease and diabetes mellitus will be seriously challenged. Here I am deeply in debt to Claude Bernard's classic philosophic work, *An Introduction to the Study of Experimental Medicine,* 1865, in which he so lucidly describes the correct uses and common abuses of *statistics* in clinical medical research. For example, the common assumption that toxemia of pregnancy is a disorder of *primiparity* has been based on statistical data which indicate that in some parts of the world and in certain socioeconomic classes, severe manifestations of this disease occur with a higher incidence in primiparous patients than in multiparous ones. The fact is neglected in such statistical analyses that even in these parts of the world and among these classes where toxemia is more common among primiparous patients, still the large majority of primiparous patients do *not* develop the disease. By thus "looking on the other side of the coin," we can immediately challenge the concept that *primiparity, per se,* has any significant *physiological* role to play in the pathogenesis of MTLP. By the same logic we can eliminate obesity, multiple pregnancy, hydramnios as *causes* of MTLP. When we consider further statistical data which indicate that MTLP has been virtually eliminated in certain areas of the world and among the upper socioeconomic classes, among women who receive good nutrition and good prenatal care, then we can further challenge the alleged role of *primiparity* as important, because certainly *primiparity* has not been eliminated in these socially advanced areas and classes.

It will be shown in this work that, contrary to popular beliefs, saluretic diuretics are *not* needed to prevent the development of MTLP during prenatal care. In fact, it will be shown that their use can be quite hazardous to women with severe manifestations of MTLP as well as being harmful to their fetuses. It will be demonstrated beyond all doubt that MTLP can be prevented without salt restriction and without great concern about "total weight gain" and obesity during pregnancy.

To both the clinical physician and his pregnant patient it should be very reassuring to learn the scientific evidence which indicates clearly that a good, well-balanced diet during pregnancy, with emphasis on high biological quality proteins, vegetables and fruits, will eliminate the threat of this serious complication. It will become obvious then that any conditions which threaten to interfere with good nutrition during pregnancy must be vigorously treated and corrected as quickly as possible. The pregnant woman can now assume the responsibility for eating a good diet when she realizes without doubt that in this way she can make the most significant contribution to her own good prenatal health and to the good health and development of her baby. The current interest and attention now focused on "weight control," obesity, salt restriction and saluretic diuretics during prenatal care can be rationally channeled into concern about well-balanced and adequate nutrition.

Armed with this scientific point of view about metabolic toxemia of late pregnancy, public health workers should be able to make more effective contributions to the problem of completely eradicating this preventable disease among women in the lower socioeconomic classes.

CHAPTER 2

CLINICAL DEFINITION AND DIFFERENTIAL DIAGNOSIS

CLINICAL DEFINITION OF METABOLIC TOXEMIA OF LATE PREGNANCY

METABOLIC TOXEMIA of late pregnancy is a disease process which occurs only associated with nonmolar pregnancy, and it is never seen in a nonpregnant female nor in a male. It is a disease whose signs develop in the latter half of pregnancy, and it subsides a few days after expulsion of the fetus and placenta. MTLP should be considered at this time a separate entity from the "toxemia syndrome" which occasionally accompanies molar pregnancy; it is an unproved and misleading assumption that these two diseases are brought about by the same underlying mechanisms, although evidence is accumulating that molar pregnancy is also caused by malnutrition.[3] A metabolically active placenta with its arteriovenous shunt effect and a growing fetus produce physiologic changes in the maternal organism quite different from those produced by a degenerating, cystic placenta usually found without a fetus in molar pregnancy.

To accurately diagnosis *uncomplicated* MTLP in any individual patient it is necessary to have made clinical observations on that patient in the first half of her pregnancy and to have found no significant signs of the disease. In clinical practice and research such observations are usually lacking because a large proportion of women with MTLP have no adequate prenatal care. A less than exact scientific diagnosis can be entertained in retrospect ten days to two weeks postpartum, for by this time all signs and symptoms of uncomplicated MTLP will have subsided.

The common *symptoms* of MTLP include headache, dizziness, visual disturbances, anorexia, nausea, vomiting, upper abdominal pain, swelling of the face and extremities and a history of acute starvation of several days duration superimposed on chronic malnutrition.

The clinical *signs* of MTLP are well described: hypertension (defined in obstetrical thinking as any pressure 140/90 mm Hg or higher recorded on two or more occasions at least six hours apart), generalized edema, proteinuria (in the absence of infection), hyperactive deep-tendon reflexes, and in the most severe cases generalized convulsions, coma, congestive heart failure with pulmonary edema, vascular collapse with hypovolemic shock and death. Signs of blood-loss shock and intra-abdominal hemorrhage associated with severe MTLP may be caused by rupture of a hemorrhagic liver.

Several standard laboratory studies are of importance in the diagnosis and management of MTLP. These include serial hematocrits, serial twenty-four-hour urinary protein loss, total serum proteins with electrophoretic separation of the albumin and globulin fractions, serum alkaline phosphatase, serum uric acid, serum urea nitrogen, fibrinogen, serum electrolytes and bromosulfophthalein retention.

In severe MTLP the serum urea nitrogen remains normal or low (except it may rise as a terminal event or after treatment with saluretic diuretics), while serum uric acid concentrations may rise to over three times normal values. Serum alkaline phosphatase may rise to over three times normal values, and fibrinogen concentrations are often double normal before any blood loss occurs. Total serum proteins may be as low as 4.0 gm% with albumin values as low as 1.2 gm% by paper-strip electrophoresis. I have observed bromosulfophthalein retentions as high as 50 percent at the end of the standard forty-five-minute test; a significant amount of both free and conjugated bromosulfophthalein may be retained.[26]

Proteinuria rarely exceeds 5.0 gm per twenty-four hours; it is often transient, fluctuating and may be minimal, even in severe MTLP. Urinary casts and blood cells are rarely found except in the terminal oliguric state or in severe dehydration. Serum electrolytes are characteristically normal in patients with severe MTLP unless they have received saluretic diuretics. CO_2 combining power of the plasma may be reduced associated with a metabolic acidosis with ketone bodies appearing in the urine.

DIFFERENTIAL DIAGNOSIS OF METABOLIC TOXEMIA OF LATE PREGNANCY

A careful clinical history must be taken in each woman suspected of having MTLP. This should include a dietary history, a careful past history for hypertension and renal disease, a socioeconomic history and a personal or psychological history. The conditions which most commonly occur in pregnant women to give rise to confusion in the diagnosis of "toxemia of pregnancy" are the following.

"ANXIETY" OR "TRANSIENT" HYPERTENSION OF EMOTIONAL STRESS. These women show hypertension (and at times hyperactive deep-tendon reflexes) as the only significant abnormal sign, have normal laboratory data and are often found to be normotensive within a few hours after delivery and sedation with morphine or other anxiety-relieving drugs. A careful psychiatric history will often reveal the nature of the emotional reaction to the stress of pregnancy. Whether these women will eventually develop so-called "essential" hypertension has yet to be learned. Such women may also have "physiologic" edema and/or proteinuria from urinary tract infection; such confusion may be very difficult to clarify except by careful study of each individual patient.

CHRONIC BENIGN "ESSENTIAL" HYPERTENSION. This occurs very commonly among Negro women of all ages in the southern states, but it is more common among women past thirty years of age.

PROTEINURIA. This is commonly caused by urinary tract infection in pregnancy, and there may be few pus cells in the urine. This is why quantitative urine cultures are so important.

"PHYSIOLOGIC EDEMA" is a common manifestation of late pregnancy in women who are otherwise perfectly normal; such edema most commonly involves the lower extremities, but moderate swelling of the hands and fingers, so that rings become tight, is frequently encountered in otherwise normal women.

RENAL DISEASES are important to consider. Glomerulonephritis (acute, subacute or chronic) is easily differentiated from MTLP (see Table II, page 65). The nephrotic syndrome (which may be caused by syphilis) is differentiated less easily, primarily by the constant, massive proteinuria which occurs in the nephrotic. Urinary loss of protein may exceed thirty grams per day in such patients. This proteinuria may persist for months and years following delivery, while proteinuria from MTLP is fluctuating from day to day and vanishes, even in the severest cases, within a week to ten days postpartum (unless complicated by renal tubular or cortical necrosis associated with prolonged shock). Renal vascular anomalies and renal neoplasms, cysts and chronic pyelonephritis may be associated with pregnancy.

DISEASES OF THE CENTRAL NERVOUS SYSTEM. Epilepsy, brain tumor, cerebrovascular accidents may occur in pregnancy to cause convulsions or coma in women who have no other signs or symptoms or laboratory data characteristic of MTLP.

MALNUTRITION *not* associated with toxic symptoms may produce hypoproteinemia and generalized edema as the only abnormalities.

It is now readily apparent that what was once considered a simple clinical problem in diagnosis is really quite complex, because MTLP may be "superimposed" on any or a combination of the above listed clinical conditions, and the unraveling of how much hypertension, proteinuria or edema is caused by MTLP and how much caused by the other associated conditions may be impossible until after delivery. Varying combinations of the above conditions in a well-nourished woman may mimic MTLP and thus lead the clinician astray.

A host of other medical diseases may be included in the differential diagnosis of MTLP: vascular anomalies such as coarctation of the aorta; congestive heart failure from other causes; malignant hypertension; hepatic diseases such as cirrhosis; and collagen diseases. The association of MTLP with poorly controlled diabetes mellitus is well established and must be kept in mind.

To those who are motivated to do research in this field, I beg a careful attention to these details of clinical differential diagnosis, for without such considerations, confusion will continue to reign. To those who must continue to manage pregnant patients until more precise biochemical knowledge becomes available, such careful differential diagnosis can only result in better and more scientific patient care. Metabolic toxemia of late pregnancy can be a lethal disease to both mother and baby; it demands our most sincere and thorough diagnostic and therapeutic skills.

CHAPTER 3

PATHOLOGY

D<small>R</small>. A<small>COSTA</small>-S<small>ISON</small>, of Manila, P.I., reported in 1936 on "A Clinicopathological Study of Eclampsia Based on Thirty-eight Autopsied Cases." *Not one* of these thirty-eight patients had had any prenatal care. Thirty-three of the thirty-eight were brought into the hospital labor unit in coma, having had convulsions at home. We learn little more of significance about the past histories of these patients from this report; we are given the autopsy findings which are so clearly the *end results* of socioeconomic neglect. The majority of these patients, as well as the majority of patients dying of eclampsia all over the world, had a hemorrhagic necrosis of the liver which is patchy, more prominent in the right lobe and in the peripheral part of the hepatic lobule.

Dr. Manuel Maqueo, of Mexico City, reported in 1964, twenty-eight years later, on fifty patients with "toxemia of pregnancy." In these women some effort was made to find out something about their nutritional background, and a direct correlation was found between a history of low protein intake and the severity of the toxemia. Needle biopsies of the liver were done in these fifty women, and thirty-eight of them showed some microscopic abnormalities.

1. Thirty-four cases showed increased von Kupffer cells.
2. Twenty-seven cases showed marked variation in size and chromatin of the nuclei of hepatic cells; many nuclei were greatly enlarged.
3. Fourteen cases showed fatty metamorphosis which was patchy in six cases, more advanced in five cases, and very marked in three cases.
4. Twelve cases showed small areas of hepatic necrosis which were more frequent in the peripheral part of the lobule. The hepatic cells were shrunken and markedly eosinophilic, and the nuclei were frequently missing.

Call and Lorentzen reported in 1965 an American Indian woman who died with a ruptured hemorrhagic and necrotic liver; she had a massive intra-abdominal hemorrhage. There is a striking color photograph of this liver in their article. A number of similar isolated cases of such liver ruptures associated with severe metabolic toxemia of late pregnancy have been reported. Unfortunately, in none of these reports do we find significant clinical data concerning the nutritional status of the patient dying of the "enigma of obstetrics."

For a number of years, then, this common pathological finding of hemorrhagic necrosis of the liver, predominantly in the right lobe and in the periportal areas microscopically, has been ignored by most clinical obstetrical authorities and passed off rather lightly as an "agonal phenomenon." Most authorities assume that the liver damage so observed is *caused* by "hypoxia," which in turn is allegedly caused by vasospasm related to the clinical hypertension. It is most important to consider that in no other recognized human disease is such a hemorrhagic necrosis of liver cells encountered. Women dying of malignant hypertension, of nephritis, of congestive heart failure, of respiratory failure, of other conditions associated with obvious "hypoxia" and hypertension, do *not* show this type of lesion. Furthermore, patients dying of acute, subacute or chronic carbon monoxide poisoning in which marked hypoxia to the peripheral tissues may result do not develop this lesion.

It will become clear as the reader grasps the basic point of view established in this book that this hepatic pathology is directly related to *malnutrition*. Pregnant women with severe metabolic toxemia of late pregnancy develop fatty and necrotic and hemorrhagic livers from *malnutrition,* not from *hypertension* nor from "hypoxia," nor from nephritis, nor from excess salt intake. This hepatic pathology is entirely preventable if the pregnant woman is able to eat, digest, absorb and metabolize all the necessary elements of nutrition for her particular pregnancy. The pregnant diabetic has a special problem in this regard as there is a tendency toward development of fatty liver in the poorly controlled, poorly nourished diabetic.

Pathology in other organs of women dying with metabolic toxemia of late pregnancy may be looked on as manifestations of injury to the endothelial cells in their peripheral vascular beds. The cause of this injury is at present unknown. There is damage to the endothelial cells in the glomerulus of the kidney nephron which results in slight swelling of the glomerulus and an increased leakage of protein. Evidence will be presented in the next chapter to indicate clearly that this renal lesion is not severe enough to cause nitrogen retention nor a significant primary reduction in glomerular filtration rate. Small hemorrhages are sometimes found in the adrenals, lungs, brain and endothelial surfaces of the heart. From present clinical and biochemical evidence I am certain that the lesions will not occur if maternal liver function is normal.

At present we have no scientific method to correlate liver pathology with liver function; therefore we must focus our primary interest and attention on biochemical and physiological studies to broaden our understanding of the pathogenesis of metabolic toxemia of late pregnancy.

CHAPTER 4

ABNORMAL PHYSIOLOGY AND BIOCHEMISTRY
HYPOVOLEMIA, HEMOCONCENTRATION, HYPOALBUMINEMIA

IT IS WELL ESTABLISHED that many patients with severe metabolic toxemia of late pregnancy develop hypovolemia with hemoconcentration evidenced clinically by a rising hematocrit. This hemoconcentration is often masked by the nutritional anemia. Several workers have demonstrated significant reduction in blood and plasma volumes in MTLP. Dieckmann clearly interpreted a rising hematocrit as a grave prognostic sign in severe toxemia, and he used hypertonic glucose solutions in varying concentrations in an attempt to correct this hemoconcentration which is usually associated with a hazardous reduction in urinary output. His results were not too satisfactory, and now we can understand why, when we recognize that the basic cause of this hypovolemia is a marked reduction in serum albumin concentration.

Although M.B. Strauss called attention to hypoproteinemia and hypovolemia in toxemia of pregnancy as early as 1935 and discussed the role of lowered serum protein colloid osmotic pressure, his work has been generally ignored by clinical obstetricians. Dieckmann was partly responsible for this, for in his classic book, *The Toxemias of Pregnancy,* in 1952, he stated: "There are no intrinsic changes in the serum proteins which might account for the edema." H.C. Mack in 1955, reporting his studies on the plasma proteins in normal and toxemic pregnancy, found a significant reduction in albumin concentration in severe toxemia. Similar studies reporting hypoalbuminemia in toxemia have emerged from all five continents.[10] The recent more accurate separation of serum protein components by electrophoresis has revealed that albumin concentrations are even lower than indicated by the older salt fractionation methods, in which some of the smaller globulins are not separated from the albumins. The significance of these low albumin levels in MTLP is further emphasized by the fact that these women have a blood volume which

[14]

may be 35 to 50 per cent reduced, and hence these are *hemoconcentrated values* which indicate clearly the marked reduction in total circulating albumin in these severely ill women.

In studying serum proteins by paper-strip electrophoresis among 500 pregnant women at Jackson Memorial Hospital, Miami, Florida, I encountered thirty toxemic women whose serum albumin concentrations were below 2.0 gm%, and these values were among the lowest seen in any patient with any disease. Patients with active cirrhosis of the liver usually had values slightly higher. The only comparable levels of albumin occurred in women with far-advanced ovarian carcinoma with peritoneal metastases who had had repeated paracenteses with removal of large quantities of protein-rich peritoneal fluid and who were eating very poorly.

A clear perception of this problem of hypovolemia associated with hypoalbuminemia will indicate to the clinician the hazards of using saluretic diuretics in these severely ill women. We can ill afford to aim our therapies blindly at the "edema." When marked generalized edema and a contracted plasma volume occur together, we must realize that these women are actually "dehydrated" into their own interstitial spaces. Any therapy which results in a further reduction of plasma volume by promoting renal excretion of water, sodium and potassium, without the concomitant mobilization of interstitial water and electrolytes, will be hazardous to these patients. Such diuretic therapy can lead to a further increase in hemoconcentration, hypovolemic shock, marked reduction in renal function associated with a serious impairment of renal blood flow and death.

Figure 16 (Chapter 6, p. 80) illustrates this clinical phenomenon clearly. After administration of intravenous chlorothiazide, this eclamptic patient developed the classical signs of hypovolemic shock with a weak, thready pulse of 140, a very narrow pulse-pressure, and sixteen hours after admission to the labor unit, she became completely anuric, cyanotic and comatose. Her response to intravenous salt-poor human serum albumin was dramatic and life-saving. Her urinary output increased to over 300 ml per hour; her pulse slowed, and the pulse-pressure widened; her edema cleared completely, and her hematocrit dropped from 43 on admission to 32 after the albumin infusions.

It is reasonable to use intravenous human serum albumin to attempt to restore the plasma colloid osmotic pressure toward normal and to correct the hypoalbuminemia. At Jackson Memorial Hospital I treated fourteen toxemic women with infusions of human serum albumin, and I observed significant diureses in thirteen of them. The patient who did not respond had a normal serum albumin concentration and minimal edema. She had received a diuretic with no response, and she delivered soon after admission and had an immediate postpartum diuresis. In none of these patients was the infusion of albumin associated with a significant rise in blood pressure, increase in pulse rate, nor with any increase in the severity of symptoms of the disease. Infusions of albumin did not appreciably increase the amount of urinary protein excreted over a twenty-four-hour period.

Case Reports

Case 1

L.F., a seventeen-year-old primigravida with no prenatal care had a convulsion at home at thirty-seven weeks gestation. She had had a poor protein intake during this pregnancy. The blood pressure was 174/124 mm; she had generalized edema. There was 2.1 gm protein in the first twenty-four-hour specimen of urine (1,600 ml). Her urinary output following 500 mgm chlorothiazide intravenously averaged 65 ml per hour for the first twenty-four hours, and during this time her hematocrit rose from 37 to 40.5. (The blood specimen sent to the lab for serum protein determinations was lost.) On the second day she was given 25 gm of human serum albumin (500 ml of a 5 per cent solution), and her urinary output immediately increased to 200 to 300 ml per hour for the next twenty-four hours, and there was total regression of clinical edema. In the second twenty-four-hour urine specimen there was only 1.7 gm of protein in 4,855 ml. The hematocrit dropped from 40.5 to 35, and the blood pressure stayed in the range of 140-150/90-100 mm.

The patient did well for the next four days and then began to show evidence of clinical edema, and the twenty-four-hour urine output dropped to 900 ml with an intake of 2800 ml. The following morning the patient was given 25 gm of albumin (500 ml of a 5 per cent solution) intravenously. By error these 500 ml were allowed to run in over a period of one hour, but there was no untoward effect. A remarkable diuresis followed with an output of

6,300 ml urine in the next twenty-four hours with an intake of 3215 ml. Her edema again disappeared.

The next day it was decided to terminate her pregnancy, and a 2,155 gm infant was delivered by Caesarean section after six days of medical therapy during which time the patient's general condition had been good. The infant did well. The patient had an uneventful postpartum course and was normotensive and without proteinuria on discharge the eighth postpartum day.

Case 2

B.B., a twenty-four-year-old primigravida with no prenatal care was admitted with severe metabolic toxemia of late pregnancy at thirty-one weeks gestation. She had had a poor protein intake during pregnancy. The blood pressure was 160/110 mm; she had generalized edema with bilateral pleural effusions and ascites. A twenty-four-hour urine specimen contained 2.8 gm of protein. The total serum proteins were 4.75 gm% with albumin 1.84 gm% and globulins 2.91 gm% by paper-strip electrophoresis. The hematocrit was 45. Following albumin infusion there was a significant diuresis with a drop in hematocrit to 33. The fetal heart tones which had been audible on admission were no longer heard on the fourth day; she went spontaneously into labor and delivered a 709 gm stillborn fetus the same day. The postpartum course was uneventful, and in the postpartum clinic four weeks later her blood pressure was 134/78 mm and there was no proteinuria.

Case 3

D.T., a seventeen-year-old primigravida at term, was admitted two hours after having had a convulsion at home. She had had no prenatal care and a poor protein intake during pregnancy. The blood pressure was 180/110 mm, and there was one-plus pitting edema of the lower extremities. The urine contained 600 mgm of protein per 100 ml. Total serum proteins were 5.72 gm% with 2.8 gm% albumin and 2.92 gm% globulins by electrophoresis.

The patient was given 500 mgm chlorothiazide intravenously, morphine sulfate and an intravenous drip of hydralazine-cryptenamine. The urinary output was only 10-15 ml per hour for the first ten hours. She was then given 10 gm of albumin (200 ml of 5 per cent solution) and two hours later 25 gm more were given. There was no improvement in urinary output; the urinary output remained at 15 ml per hour. The patient went spontaneously into labor and with oxytocin stimulation was delivered of an infant weighing 3248 gm who did well. Delivery occurred twenty-three hours after admission; the patient put out 4520 ml urine during the first day and had an uneventful postpartum course.

Case 4

B.C., a twenty-six-year-old gravida 2, para 1, was admitted to our hospital at thirty-three weeks gestation having had no prenatal care. The patient had had a poor intake of protein during pregnancy. Wasting of skeletal muscles had been present as long as she could remember; the diagnosis of myotonia dystrophica was made by our medical consultants. She had marked generalized edema. The blood pressure was 140/100 mm; a twenty-four-hour urine contained 2.1 gm protein. Total serum proteins were 5.8 gm% with 1.86 gm% albumin and 4.0 gm% globulins; the serum urea nitrogen was 16 mgm%.

The patient was put on a low salt diet and given 25 mgm hydrochlorothiazide by mouth daily for nine days. Her appetite remained poor and she ate little. She developed a low-salt syndrome with serum urea nitrogen rising to 57 mgm%. This improved with addition of salt to her diet and the discontinuance of the diuretic. A repeat serum protein study revealed serum proteins to have dropped to 4.99 gm% with 1.7 gm% albumin and 3.26 gm%globulins. The urinary protein output per twenty-four hours increased to 4.0 gm.

Three weeks after admission the total serum proteins had fallen to 4.47 gm% with serum albumin of 1.54 gm%. At this time it was first observed that the patient was developing hydramnios with a 4 cm increase in fundal height over a twenty-four-hour period, and the fetal parts became hard to outline.

The urinary output averaged 50 ml per hour for twelve hours, and then she was given 37.5 gm of albumin (25 per cent solution) intravenously, and the urinary output increased to 150 ml per hour for the next twelve hours. The following day she received 37.5 gm albumin intravenously with a similar increase in output to 150 ml per hour for twelve hours. The next day the patient went spontaneously into labor and was delivered of a normal 2480 gm infant who did well. Her urinary output on the day of delivery was 3775 ml with an intake of 1600 ml. She had an uneventful postpartum course, and four weeks later had no evidence of hypertension nor of proteinuria.

Case 5

M.U., a twenty-one-year-old primigravida, was admitted with severe toxemia at thirty-eight weeks gestation having had no pre-natal care. She had just arrived in Florida from Cuba. She had had a poor protein intake during pregnancy. The blood pressure was 190/100 mm; there were marked generalized edema and hyperactive deep-tendon reflexes. The first twenty-four-hour urine contained 3.2 gm protein. The total serum proteins were 5.10 with 1.85 gm% albumin and 3.25 gm% globulins. The hematocrit was 32.

Following 250 mgm chlorothiazide intravenously, the first twen-ty-four-hour output was less than 50 ml per hour (1100 ml); she was given then two 25 gm infusions of albumin (25 per cent solution), and her urine output increased to 200 ml per hour for three hours following each infusion; the total twenty-four-hour urine output rose to 2600 ml, and there was appreciable clearing of clinical edema.

Labor began spontaneously eight days after admission, and she was delivered of an infant weighing 2750 gm who did well. Blood loss was normal at delivery, but on the second postpartum day the hematocrit had dropped from 32 to 23.5. She was treated with ferrous sulfate. She was discharged on the seventh post-partum day with a normal blood pressure and a trace of protein remaining in the urine.

The cause of this hypoalbuminemia in metabolic toxemia of late pregnancy is not known at present. From my own observations in many severely toxic and malnourished women whose serum albumin levels fell off rapidly over a few days associated with a marked in-crease of generalized edema, I suspect that impairment in hepatic synthesis of albumin plays a major role. It must be kept in mind that there is an "exchangeable albumin pool" of 250 to 300 gm in the body tissues and that the tissues actively metabolize 15 to 20 gm of albumin daily.[13] In these toxemic women with poor nutrition be-fore and during pregnancy, it is reasonable to suspect that this pool may be depleted; hence it will be difficult to maintain adequate serum concentrations except by repeated infusions. This is exactly my ex-perience; the infused albumin leaves the circulation in a few hours. Serum albumin has other important physiological functions beside those of maintaining plasma volume; it contributes to the buffering capacity of the plasma and its functions to bind various hormones, ions and toxins. Its use in severe MTLP thus has further strong theoretical support.

The improvement in renal function as evidenced by increase in urinary output which begins immediately following albumin infusions and/or delivery in women with severe MTLP is a very important physiologic phenomenon to study, for it gives a strong indication that the glomerular endothelial lesion is *not* of *primary functional significance* in the development of oliguria and generalized edema in these women. Delivery removes the arteriovenous shunt effect of the intervillous space so that the blood which previously had been shunted through the placental site now becomes available for systemic and renal flow. Delivery is analagous to a transfusion of blood or plasma causing immediate expansion of the blood volume. Each gram of infused albumin can mobilize 20 ml of interstitial fluid. When renal blood flow is thus increased by expanding the plasma volume, *the toxemic kidneys function.*

An observation made in Case 4 above is of considerable interest: The patient's serum albumin concentration was observed to drop from 1.86 gm% to 1.54 gm% over a three-week period while she was being treated for toxemia in the hospital. She developed acute hydramnios which was definitely *preceded* by her toxemia and not its *cause.* This suggests that hypoalbuminemia may play some role in the pathogenesis of acute hydramnios associated with MTLP. Since the fetus of the toxemic woman usually has a much higher serum level of albumin than the mother,[14] the question arises: Does the colloid osmotic pressure gradient across the fetal capillary play a significant role in transfer of water and electrolytes to the fetus? Significant lowering of the maternal plasma colloid osmotic pressure will produce an increase in transfer of water and electrolytes into the fetal circulation and a decrease in absorption of amniotic fluid across the amnion-chorionic membranes. If the fetus has normal renal function, this would result in an increase of fluid within the amniotic sac. Further studies and observations are required to answer these questions. In 1960, Buckingham at Northwestern Medical School published clinical data on patients with hydramnios which suggest there are two distinct mechanisms for development of hydramnios: fetal and maternal. Those women with maternal complications associated with hydramnios (toxemia, diabetes mellitus, Rh sensitization) had no congenitally deformed infants in his series. Among the mothers who gave birth to congenitally deformed infants associated with hydramnios, *there was no toxemia.*

Dr. Shioichi Sato of Keio University, Tokyo, Japan, has reported diureses and improvement in the clinical condition of toxemic women following the infusion of dextran and other plasma-expanders. He has come to realize the importance of hypovolemia and hypoalbuminemia in toxemia independently and has held this subject worthy of study and therapy. He wrote me from Japan recently: "You are one of the first persons in the whole world to agree with many of my ideas." I wrote back and told him that I know how he feels.

HEPATIC DYSFUNCTION

While many authorities agree that significant liver dysfunction exists in severe metabolic toxemia of late pregnancy, they do not accept the altered hepatic function as playing any significant role in the pathogenesis of the disease process. They do not consider that the hepatic dysfunction is *caused* by malnutrition but rather that it is the end result of the disease and caused by "hypoxia" to the hepatic cells. As previously discussed (Chap. 1), there is no evidence that such "hypoxia" exists in MTLP. The strongest evidence I can advance at the present for the primary role of malnutrition leading to hepatic dysfunction is presented in the subsequent sections of this chapter on the treatment of patients with mild MTLP with neomycin and a high protein diet and in the data in Chapter 8, which clearly establishes that this disease can be totally prevented by good prenatal nutrition. Furthermore, I have made many clinical observations of patients who were put on starvation diets by their physicians for obesity early in pregnancy, and this led directly to their developing metabolic toxemia of late pregnancy. Therefore I am convinced that the basic metabolic abnormality in MTLP lies within hepatic cells and that this altered hepatic metabolism is in turn directly caused by poor prenatal nutrition.

I am presenting here a viewpoint at odds with the currently accepted ideas, because I look upon *vasoconstriction* as merely a clinical manifestation or *end result* of a metabolic hepatic disease of nutritional deficiency. The symptoms of severe MTLP are the symptoms of liver disease: anorexia, nausea; vomiting; malaise; and epigastric pain. The pathological findings of fatty infiltration and hemorrhagic necrosis of the hepatic cells with an occasionally reported case of frank rupture of the liver with hematoperitoneum are compatible with this concept. The clear-cut association of MTLP with poverty and inadequate prenatal care likewise substantiates this point of view. It is generally agreed that in the private practice of obstetrics here in the United States the incidence of this disease is 1 per cent or less, while in certain economically depressed areas of our nation and in certain underprivileged groups the incidence may be thirty-five times higher. We can no longer ignore the scientific evidence of the important roles of malnutrition and hepatic dysfunction in the pathogenesis of metabolic toxemia of late pregnancy.

Impairment in Steroid Metabolism

As pregnancy advances toward term, the placental production of steroids, estrogens and progesterone increases. It has recently been learned that the placenta secretes about 300 mgm of progesterone daily during the last few weeks of pregnancy; one patient with twins has been observed to secrete 520 mgm of progesterone in a twenty-four-hour period.[17] Obviously this puts an increased load on the hepatic enzyme systems which metabolize these steroids. Steroids with alcoholic groups are conjugated within hepatic cells primarily with uridine diphosphate glucuronic acid via a glucuronyl transferase enzyme system; a smaller part is conjugated with sulfate.[18] The steps in metabolism of progesterone in the pregnant woman may be taken as a model for other steroids' metabolism (Fig. A).

1. Progesterone is produced by the trophoblasts of the placenta and secreted into the maternal blood in the intervillous space.
2. It is bound to a transfer protein and carried to the liver.
3. It is taken up by the hepatic cells.
4. Within hepatic cells: (a) Progesterone is reduced by the addition of hydrogen atoms to *pregnanediol;* (b) Pregnanediol is conjugated with uridine diphosphate glucuronic acid to pregnanediol glucuronide via a glucuronyl transferase enzyme sys-

PROGESTERONE METABOLISM IN PREGNANCY

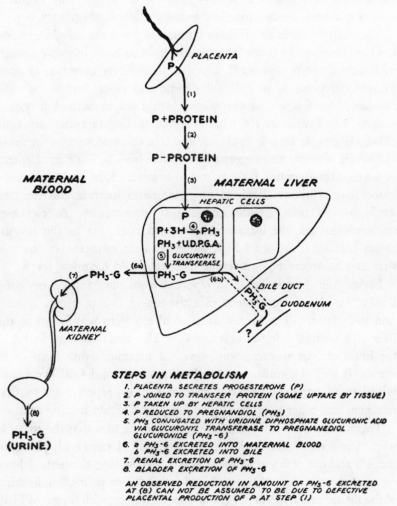

STEPS IN METABOLISM

1. PLACENTA SECRETES PROGESTERONE (P)
2. P JOINED TO TRANSFER PROTEIN (SOME UPTAKE BY TISSUE)
3. P TAKEN UP BY HEPATIC CELLS
4. P REDUCED TO PREGNANDIOL (PH₃)
5. PH₃ CONJUGATED WITH URIDINE DIPHOSPHATE GLUCURONIC ACID VIA GLUCURONYL TRANSFERASE TO PREGNANEDIOL GLUCURONIDE (PH₃-G)
6. a PH₃-G EXCRETED INTO MATERNAL BLOOD
   b PH₃-G EXCRETED INTO BILE
7. RENAL EXCRETION OF PH₃-G
8. BLADDER EXCRETION OF PH₃-G

AN OBSERVED REDUCTION IN AMOUNT OF PH₃-G EXCRETED AT (8) CAN NOT BE ASSUMED TO BE DUE TO DEFECTIVE PLACENTAL PRODUCTION OF P AT STEP (1)

Figure A. See Fruton and Simmonds: *General Biochemistry,* Chapter 26, Chemistry and Metabolism of Steroids.

tem; and (c) Pregnanediol glucuronide is then excreted from the hepatic cells—part going into the bile and part back into the maternal blood via the hepatic veins.

5. Pregnanediol glucuronide is then carried to the maternal kidneys and excreted in the urine.

It becomes obvious that estimations of the amount of pregnanediol glucuronide excreted in a twenty-four-hour urine can only begin to answer questions about progesterone metabolism in pregnancy.

The twenty-four-hour urinary excretion of pregnanediol glucuronide has been observed by many investigators to be reduced in many women with toxemia of pregnancy.[19] Likewise the urinary excretion of conjugated estrogens, as well as aldosterone and other adrenal steroids, has been found lower in toxemic women than in normal pregnant women.[19, 21] Frantz in 1960 has reported finding *increased* amounts of 6-OH-cortisol, the principal *unconjugated* corticosteroid, in the urine of toxemic women, and suggested that there may be some impairment in the usual conjugation mechanisms in toxemia. Eton and Short have found normal plasma levels of progesterone in toxemia and elevated levels in twin, twin toxemic and diabetic pregnancies. A few cases scattered through the literature have been confusing to the investigators because they found high blood levels of estrogens in toxemic women who according to popular theories should have low levels.

Parker and Tenney in 1938 reported from the Mallory Institute, Boston, on the tissue content of estrogens in five pregnant women and their fetuses. The largest amount of estrogens was found in the liver of a woman dying of eclampsia; smaller amounts were found in the livers of four women, who were not toxemic, dying from other causes. It was of significance that both maternal and fetal livers contained more estrogens than the placentas. This report suggests that estrogens and other steroids may be "trapped" within hepatic cells.

There is more clinical evidence supporting the idea that the toxemic woman is actually overloaded in the majority of cases with placental steroids and not deficient in them as has been so long thought. I have on several occasions observed the so-called "liver palms," a flushing of the thenar and hypothenar eminences, in women with severe MTLP, and in several such women I have observed spider angiomas. Also I have seen several infants born to toxemic women show marked hypertrophy of the breasts. It seems highly unlikely that these women were deficient in progesterone and estrogens. I have also occasionally seen a Pap smear report on a toxemic woman returned with the note: "excessive estrogen effect." The "ripening" of the cervix occurs earlier in many toxemic women so that they frequently go into spontaneous labor prematurely. It is a well known clinical fact among obstetricians who treat a large number of toxemic women that their labors can usually be induced relatively easily before term. This "ripening" or preparation of the cervix for delivery is thought to be enhanced by the placental steroid hormones.

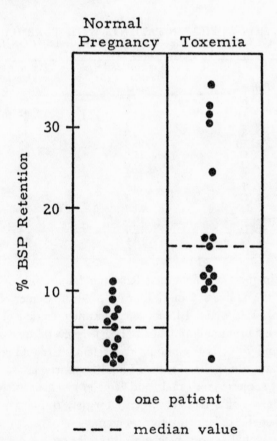

FIGURE B. BSP retention in fifteen normal pregnant patients in the third trimester and fifteen toxemic patients.

Another related subject requires clarification. It is true that some women with severe MTLP have small placentas with large infarcted areas which cause their fetuses to fail to grow normally, and such women probably have a below normal production of placental progesterone and estrogens. However, the majority of women with MTLP do *not* have such small infarcted placentas; and on the other side of the coin, the majority of women with infarcted, small placentas associated with small, malnourished infants do *not* have MTLP.[25] These observations suggest that infarcted placentas may be the *result* of MTLP but are not its *cause.*

TABLE I
BSP RETENTION IN FIFTEEN PATIENTS WITH TOXEMIA OF LATE PREGNANCY WITH PER CENT OF RETAINED BSP-CONJUGATED METABOLITES

Patient	Per cent BSP retention at 45 minutes	Per cent of conjugated metabolites
B. L.	37.4	62
L. Y.	33.4	42
B. L.	32.5	32
D. E.	32.0	36
T. H.	25.3	43
G. O.	17.0	80
J. M.	17.0	54
D. R.	15.8	55
N. T.	13.4	80
C. C.	12.0	55
L. D.	12.0	25
G. G.	10.6	49
R. D.	10.4	24
B. E.	10.4	39
R. B.	2.0	

Working in the Gastrointestinal Research Laboratory of Dr. John Carbone at the University of California Medical Center, San Francisco, Virginia Hjelte and I found a significant retention of both free and conjugated bromosulfophthalein (BSP) in several toxemic women after the standard forty-five-minute dye retention test (Fig. B Table I). These data are similar to those found by Carbone and Hjelte in nonpregnant subjects, both male and female, given progesterone and other steroids and offer indirect evidence for the "trapping" of steroids within the hepatic cells in toxemic women.

It is obvious that further biochemical studies on the metabolism of steroids in toxemic and normal pregnancy are indicated to fill in the details, but I am convinced from present biochemical and clinical evidence that a significant impairment in hepatic conjugation of these steroids exists in toxemic women and plays a significant role in the pathogenesis of the disease. In fact, this is one of the reasons that MTLP is not encountered in other nutritional deficiency syndromes in the nonpregnant; one of the unique physiologic and biochemical facts of pregnancy is the presence in the body of a large endocrine organ, the placenta, which is capable of producing large quantities of steroid hormones—and then is removed quickly at delivery. In a personal communication, R. V. Short described to me how quickly the blood levels of progesterone fall after delivery so that in many cases he was unable to detect progesterone in the maternal plasma five minutes after delivery of the placenta.

I suspect that sodium-retaining steroids having their effect on the renal tubules play an important role in the sodium and water retention seen in women who develop clinical edema in pregnancy yet have normal serum protein levels.

Impairment in Detoxication of Other Aromatic Compounds

Another important source of physiologically active compounds which are detoxified by hepatic cells is the lower gastrointestinal tract. Here bacterial enzymes working on certain aromatic amino acids produce various amines, phenol, cresols, and other by-products (as well as ammonia) which are absorbed and carried to the liver via the portal vein. Some of these aromatic alcoholic compounds are conjugated with glucuronic acid and sulfate and hence may retard steroid conjugation by competitive inhibition. In severe cases of malnutrition they may accumulate within hepatic cells and cause death of the cell. The amines are detoxified by amine oxidases. These compounds are believed to play a role in the pathogenesis of hepatic coma.

The value of intestinal antisepsis in the management of hepatic coma, impending coma and in portal systemic shunts has been well established since 1955. We have thus a precedent from internal medicine: *If* the liver begins to fail in its function of detoxication, the lower gastrointestinal tract *can* become the source of toxic compounds capable of causing damage to the body. The reduction in smooth muscle tone and the crowding of the gastrointestinal tract by the expanding uterus produce a unique situation in pregnancy in which constipation is notorious and the opportunities enhanced for absorption of these potentially toxic compounds. The often observed pathological finding that the toxemic lesions of hemorrhagic necrosis predominate in the *right* lobe of the liver suggested to me that these GI compounds may play some role in this cellular damage because of the streamlining of blood from the lower GI tract into the right lobe via the portal vein. This is mere speculation. Other explanations of differences in metabolism of peripheral hepatic cells have been advanced, such as the differences in blood supply related to the hepatic arterial and portal circulations.

The following compounds, all arising in the gastrointestinal tract, and all detoxified primarily in the liver, have been reported to be present in abnormal or increased quantities in the serum or urine of patients with toxemia of pregnancy: tyramine; indican; indole; and serotonin.[27] The Krupps in 1960 concluded from their studies of serotonin in toxemia of pregnancy: "There is no reason to postulate increased serotonin production in the eclamptogenic toxemias, but rather it would seem more likely that in some instances its detoxication is delayed or inhibited." Serotonin is detoxified primarily in the liver cells by an amine oxidase system. It is not possible to implicate any one of these compounds as producing signs or symptoms of MTLP, but the fact that they appear in the serum or urine in increased quantities is further evidence that the hepatic detoxication enzyme systems of toxemic women are overloaded and/or impaired.

Miale and I reported in 1961 from Jackson Memorial Hospital, Miami, Florida, some evidence compatible with the idea that impairment in glucuronic acid conjugation of aromatic compounds is present in toxemic women compared with normal women. We gave anisic acid (p-methoxybenzoic acid) by mouth and intravenously to normal and toxemic pregnant women in the third trimester and

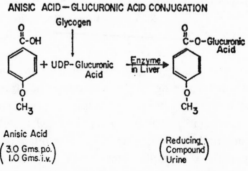

ANISIC ACID — GLUCURONIC ACID CONJUGATION

FIGURE 1. Conjugation of uridine diphosphate glucuronic acid with anisic acid.

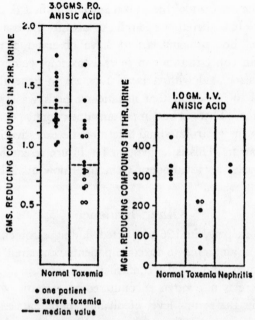

FIGURE 2. Anisic conjugation in normal and toxemic pregnancy. *At left*: after 3.0 gm per os; *At right*: after 1.0 gm IV.

found a significant reduction in urinary excretion of glucuronic acid in the toxemic woman. A limitation of this study was admitted: We did not measure renal clearance of the metabolized anisic acid. However, in two women with nephritis and elevated serum urea nitrogen levels we found normal excretions of the glucuronic acid metabolite, and all the toxemic women tested had adequate urinary outputs (greater than 50 ml per hour) and normal or low serum urea nitrogen concentrations (Figs. 1 & 2).

Hypoalbuminemia

This has been discussed above. It is not scientifically established that the low serum levels of albumin in toxemic women are *caused* by impairment in hepatic synthesis of albumin. It is clear that the low levels cannot be explained by urinary loss (as in nephrosis), for I have observed many women with insignificant urinary loss of albumin in the urine who had very low serum levels. Electrophoretic separation of the urinary proteins in these women with MTLP often reveals that the majority of their proteinuria is in fact due to excretion of globulins. (It is therefore scientific to discard the use of the term, "albuminuria," for proteinuria.) I have observed a rapid fall in serum albumin concentrations in several toxemic women over a few days period associated with a rapid increase in generalized edema; this suggested to my mind that hepatic synthesis was falling behind tissue utilization. There is one important unexplored possibility: Loss of albumin in the gastrointestinal tract may be excessive in these mal-nourished women. This is a question for future research and should be quickly resolved with modern techniques now available for study of protein metabolism.

Other Evidence

Krauss, of Leipzig, in 1961 reported finding significant elevations of whole blood ammonia in toxemic patients compared with normal pregnant women, and I have confirmed this in a small group of six patients. There is also often encountered in toxemic women a significant rise in the serum level of alkaline phosphatase activity and also a marked rise in fibrinogen concentrations. Part of this increase in alkaline phosphatase and fibrinogen levels may be associated with hemoconcentration.

ANEMIA

A microcytic, iron deficiency, nutritional-type anemia is frequently encountered in patients with MTLP. A macrocytic, folic acid deficiency anemia has also been reported in quite a number of women with this disease. Both types of anemia, which may occur together in the same patient, reflect the poor nutritional status of the toxemic woman. I think the principal factor which has blocked real understanding of the significance of hypovolemia, hemoconcentration and hypoalbuminemia as discussed above is the fact that this commonly associated anemia *masks* the hemoconcentration. Case 5 reported above is a typical example, in that her hematocrit reading dropped from 32 to 23.5 after delivery; it is a common experience on the postpartum wards of our city-county hospitals to find that the toxemic patient turns up with a severe anemia on the third or fourth postpartum day (with no history of excessive blood loss at delivery). This problem of anemia is completely preventable with good prenatal care, good prenatal nutrition, and iron and folic acid supplementation whenever necessary.

SERUM URIC ACID AND SERUM UREA NITROGEN

It has been long observed that in severe MTLP there is retention of uric acid in the serum, and this is related in part to a reduction in renal excretion of uric acid. The basic biochemistry is obscure to me. I have seen serum uric concentrations as high as 20 mgm% in severely toxemic women with normal serum concentrations of urea nitrogen. This is, in fact, characteristic of MTLP: a normal or low serum urea nitrogen level associated with a higher than normal uric acid level. The urinary excretion of urea nitrogen is often quite low in women with MTLP; I have observed a twenty-four-hour excretion of urea nitrogen as low as 0.7 gm. This is clearly evidence of a protein-deficient diet, because when these patients receive an adequate intake of protein after admission to the hospital, it is possible to observe a rise in both serum urea nitrogen and in the twenty-four-hour urinary excretion of urea nitrogen. During many years experience with attention to this question, I have not observed an abnormally high concentration of serum urea nitrogen in a patient with MTLP except after treatment with saluretic diuretics or in a terminal state of oliguria. As mentioned in Chapter 2, the serum urea nitrogen concentration is of considerable value in differentiating MTLP from glomerulonephritis occurring in the last half of pregnancy (Table II, p. 65).

ACIDOSIS

In many patients admitted with severe MTLP it is possible to obtain a history of several days of acute starvation (including nausea and vomiting) superimposed on chronic malnutrition. This is associated with a reduction in the carbon dioxide-combining power of the plasma, a metabolic acidosis; there may be ketones in the urine. The poorly controlled, poorly nourished diabetic often presents herself with severe acidosis associated with MTLP, and this must always be kept in mind. Hepatic glycogen is depleted in these patients and their hepatic cells may be infiltrated with fat. It is obvious that these patients require fluids to combat dehydration, and they need glucose and protein to combat starvation and to replenish hepatic glycogen.

It is a common clinical mistake to limit fluid intake on toxemic women and to keep them without oral intake for several days.

"RAT ECLAMPSIA"

Hemorrhagic necrosis of the liver has been studied in malnourished, protein-depleted rats for many years by Himsworth, Paul György, Glynn and others. They found that rats on a very low protein diet (torula yeast) were protected from this liver necrosis by methionine, vitamin E, selenium and cystine, which would protect them from dying in coma with such an associated hemorrhagic necrosis of the liver. Recently, Donald McKay at Columbia has been working with pregnant rats fed a low protein, high oxidized fat diet, and he has observed a similar hemorrhagic necrosis of the liver as well as abruptions of the placenta and generalized endothelial damage with hemorrhages in the lungs, adrenals, etc. These lesions are very similar to those encountered in women dying of metabolic toxemia of late pregnancy. The question arises: Is the disease which McKay is producing in pregnant rats fed a low protein, high fat diet the same disease encountered in pregnant women on low protein, high fat diets, namely metabolic toxemia of late pregnancy? (The constant scientific problem facing us when we work with experimental animals on a disease of unknown etiology in humans is the question of whether what we do to the animal to produce abnormality is the same thing that is happening to our human patients before they present themselves to us as "cases" of a clinical disease entity.) I think the scientific evidence is clear in this case and that these two processes are the same, and that McKay's model is a valuable laboratory tool in working out many unsolved biochemical problems of MTLP. The reasons for this opinion may be simply stated.

1. Women who develop severe MTLP in our southern states among our lowest socioeconomic class have diets which *are* low in protein and high in fat.

2. I have observed ten obese pregnant women who developed MTLP while on physician-prescribed starvation diets during their prenatal course. (This suggests that the presence of high fat content in the diet is not necessary for development of MTLP.)

3. McKay and others have observed that neomycin and other "nonabsorbable" antibiotics prevent 75 per cent of the animals from dying of the disease. I have observed beneficial effects of similar intestinal sterilization in a number of *toxemic women,* whose case reports are presented in the next section.

ROLE OF THE GASTROINTESTINAL BACTERIAL FLORA IN THE PATHOGENESIS OF METABOLIC TOXEMIA OF LATE PREGNANCY

The rational for my clinical study on the effects of high protein diets and sterilization of the gastrointestinal tract in women with MTLP has been discussed above under hepatic dysfunction. To encourage other clinical obstetricians to confirm or discredit my data, I include the following "protocol" which is designed to guide such studies. (It can be modified to study each factor separately.)

Protocol for High Protein Diet, Bowel Sterilization Study in Metabolic Toxemia of Late Pregnancy

I. *Theory*

Epidemiologic, clinical and biochemical studies point to protein malnutrition as playing an important role in the pathogenesis of MTLP. Malnutrition can lead to liver dysfunction, and there is evidence that the liver is grossly damaged in severe MTLP. Functional impairment is reflected in hypoalbuminemia, elevation of alkaline phosphatase, elevation in plasma fibrinogen and deficiency in hepatic detoxication enzyme systems. As pregnancy advances, the placenta produces an increasing quantity of steroids which the liver must conjugate and excrete.

A number of aromatic compounds arise in the lower GI tract from bacterial enzymatic degradation of amino acids; phenols; cresols; indole; tyramine; phenylethylamine. Ammonia is also formed. These compounds are absorbed and carried to the liver via the portal vein. Here the aromatic alcohols and acids are conjugated with glucuronic acid and sulfate, the same substrates used to conjugate steroids, while the amines are oxidized by amine oxidases.

Acute and chronic malnutrition can deplete both enzymes and substrates needed to handle the increased load on the detoxication systems brought on by pregnancy. During pregnancy there is increased need for protein to supply the growing fetus and to increase maternal protein stores for lactation to follow.

It seems reasonable to reduce the GI bacterial flora in MTLP in an effort to reduce the quantity of compounds competing for detoxication in the liver. A high protein diet is important to maintain the protein reserves in the liver upon which the detoxication systems depend, as well as to supply the increased maternal and fetal needs of pregnancy.

II. *Choice of Patients*

1. Metabolic toxemia of late pregnancy—thirty-eight weeks or less gestation.
2. Patient not in labor—membranes intact.
3. Patient able to take medications and food by mouth.
4. No evidence of fetal distress—fetal heart tones present and normal.

III. *Initial Lab Studies*

1. Routine CBC, urinalysis, serology, Rh and type as indicated.
2. Blood chemistries: serum urea nitrogen; serum uric acid; creatinine; alkaline phosphatase; total serum proteins with electrophoretic separation of albumin and globulins; BSP retention.
3. Twenty-four hour urine for total protein, urea nitrogen and total sulfur.

IV. *Plan of Initial Hospital Management*

1. Regular diet with no sodium restriction (for three to five days while initial observations are made and lab studies evaluated).
2. Full ambulation—encourage patient to stay active out of bed.
3. Check fetal heart tones, blood pressure q six hours and record on graphic sheet.
4. Weigh daily and record on graphic sheet.
5. Mild analgesics and phenobarbital 15 to 30 mgm q 6 h if needed.
6. Nausea, vomiting, bowel movements to be charted as well as how well the patient is eating her diet.
7. Twenty-four-hour urine collected daily under toluene for protein—send aliquot to lab daily.
8. Physician to measure fundal height daily.
9. No diuretic drugs, no sodium restriction, no anti-hypertensive medication.
10. Explain study to patient and obtain her permission and co-operation.

V. *Plan of Subsequent Hospital Management*
1. Neomycin sulfate 0.5 gm tab—tabs 2 q 4 h. for three days and then tabs 2 q 6 h.
2. Record number, volume and consistency of stools and instruct patient to collect urine and stool separately.
3. Three days after neomycin started, patient is to begin 2200 cal, 120 gm protein diet with no sodium restriction.
4. If patient goes into labor, she is to receive 5 mgm Vit. K IM before going into labor unit.
5. If patient or fetus at any time seem to be in hazardous condition, study will be discontinued and delivery effected as quickly as possible.
6. If there is no clinical improvement in two weeks, neomycin will be discontinued and regular classical therapy instituted.
7. If clinical improvement is observed, neomycin will be discontinued after one week, and patient will be observed for another week or until recurrence of signs or symptoms of MTLP.
8. When signs or significant symptoms of MTLP recur, neomycin will be restarted and management followed as above.
9. Neomycin will be discontinued when labor begins and not restarted.
10. Patient will be continued on full ambulation and encouraged to be active out of bed doing chores about ward when possible if she is willing.

From February, 1960, to February, 1962, while a resident in the Department of Obstetrics-Gynecology, University of Miami School of Medicine, at Jackson Memorial Hospital, Miami, Florida, I treated ten toxemic patients essentially as outlined above with a few variations. I started out originally with both neomycin and sulfathalidine as outlined by Poth as the most effective method to completely suppress the GI bacterial flora. Since the detailed case reports of these patients have not been published elsewhere, I include them here along with three "controls," patients with mild toxemia who were not given antibiotics to suppress the GI bacterial flora.

Case Reports

Case 1, M.F.
Hx: Twenty-eight-year-old gravida 4 para 3 of thirty-five weeks

gestation was admitted February 12, 1960, with complaints of nausea, vomiting, abdominal pain and severe headaches for three days. She was acutely intoxicated with alcohol. She had gained no weight during this pregnancy and had no edema. Her diet had been low in protein throughout pregnancy. Her husband had been killed in a barroom brawl the preceding summer. On three visits to a county clinic in the second trimester of this pregnancy she had been normotensive and without proteinuria.

P.E.: Blood pressure 144/94 mm; weight 118 lbs. Eyegrounds showed acute hypertensive changes, Grade I. Estimated fetal weight was 2400 gm. There was no edema of the extremities. Deep-tendon reflexes were normal.

Lab Data: Hematocrit 33. Urine protein in twenty-four-hours: negative. Serum uric acid 9.8 mgm%. Serum urea nitrogen 3.0 mgm%. Total serum proteins 6.51 gm% with 2.62 gm% albumin and 3.89 gm% globulins. Alk. Phosphatase 8.6 Bodansky Units (4 units upper limit of normal). One twenty-four-hour urinary excretion of catechol amines was normal. A twenty-four-hour urinary excretion of urea nitrogen was 1.5 gm. Quantitative urine culture was negative.

Hospital Course (Fig. 3):

The patient remained nauseated and vomited several times and ate nothing for about three days and received intravenous fluids.

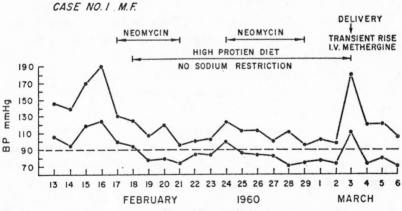

FIGURE 3. Response to high protein diet and bowel sterilization. Poorly nourished woman with three children and no husband. She had gained no weight during pregnancy and had no edema but marked hypertension.

Her blood pressure went up to 170/120 on February 15, 1960, the third hospital day, and to 190/124 on February 16, when she had a profuse nosebleed. She was treated this day with an intravenous drip of hydralazine-cryptenamine, pentobarbital, magnesium sulfate, hydrochlorothiazide and morphine; her blood pressure came down to 140/100 after three hours.

The next day her blood pressure was 130/100; all medications were discontinued, and she was started on neomycin and Vitamin K. On February 18 she began the high protein diet (120 gm protein, 2200 cal) and received an injection of Imferon. She was ambulatory and had no sodium restriction. After forty-eight hours her blood pressure was normal. She received neomycin for five days and then it was stopped. Her headaches cleared and her appetite was good. Her weight was stable.

Three days later she developed headache and her blood pressure returned to 100 mm diastolic and remained in the range 90-100 mm for over twelve hours; she was started back on neomycin. Her blood pressure returned to normal within twenty-four hours and remained normal until March third when she began spontaneous labor. Throughout her labor, which lasted six hours, her blood pressure and deep-tendon reflexes remained normal. She had a spontaneous obstetrical delivery of a 2070 gm female infant who did well. Immediately postpartum she was given 0.2 mgm methyl ergonovine intravenously, and her blood pressure went up immediately to 180/110; she was given 15 mgm morphine sulfate intramuscularly right away, and the blood pressure dropped to 110/82 in thirty minutes after injection and remained normal throughout her postpartum course. She was discharged on the fourth day in good condition.

Case 2, V.A.

Hx: Nineteen-year-old gravida 3 para 2 was admitted April 19, 1960, at approximately thirty-eight weeks gestation with the chief complaint of abdominal pain, dizziness and swelling of feet and legs for three weeks. She had no prenatal care. Her weight gain by history was 50 lbs during this pregnancy. She had had two previous term deliveries with no evidence of toxemia. She had had a poor protein intake during this pregnancy. She was unmarried and lived in a large family.

P.E.: Obese nineteen-year-old female with marked edema of face, hands and lower extremities. Blood pressure was 150/100. Eyegrounds were normal. Estimated fetal weight was 3400 gm. Extremities showed a four-plus pitting edema above the knees and also edema of hands and fingers. Deep-tendon reflexes were normal.

Lab Data: Hematocrit: 34. Urine protein in twenty-four hours: negative. Serum uric acid: 7 mgm%. Serum urea nitrogen: 6.2 mgm%. Total serum proteins: 5.49 gm% with albumin 2.07 gm%. Alkaline phosphatase: 3.1 BU. A twenty-four-hour urine excretion of urea nitrogen was 1.4 gm. (After two

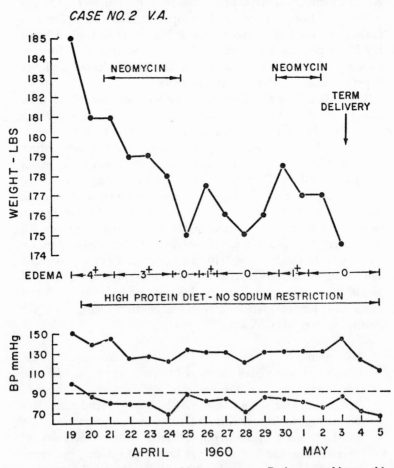

FIGURE 4. Mild metabolic toxemia of late pregnancy. Patient gave history of low protein intake during pregnancy. She lost 10½ lbs before delivery with no dietary salt restriction, no diuretic, and full ambulation. Edema reaccumulated when neomycin was discontinued and disappeared when it was restarted.

weeks on the high protein diet, the total serum proteins had risen from 5.49 to 6.47 gm%, and the albumin from 2.07 to 2.52 gm%.) A quantitative urine culture was negative.

Hospital Course: The patient received only one dose of Dilantin 100 mgm and morphine sulfate 8.0 mgm intramuscularly on admission and no other medication except ferrous sulfate, the bowel prep and Vit. K. Her weight stabilized at 181 lbs after two days, and she was started on neomycin and the high protein diet. Her blood pressure remained normal after twenty-four hours, and she had a significant diuresis, losing to 175 (6 lbs) in five days with the disappearance of all her edema (Fig. 4).

The neomycin was stopped, and she did well for five days and then showed a reappearance of edema and a 2½ lb gain in twenty-four hours with a rise in blood pressure to 130/86. She was started back on neomycin and lost from 178½ to 174½ in the next four days.

On May 2 she began to leak amniotic fluid and was induced with intravenous pitocin drip after twenty-four hours. Her blood pressure and deep tendon reflexes remained normal throughout labor and delivery. She had a postpartum hemorrhage from uterine atony and was given 1500 ml whole blood. Her postpartum course was otherwise normal and she was discharged on the third day with blood pressure of 110/70 and hemoglobin of 11.3 gm.

Case 3, Q.O.

Hx: Thirty-four-year-old gravida 7 para 6 was admitted February 17, 1961, at thirty-eight weeks gestation with no prenatal care. By history she had gained 42 lbs (167 to 209) and had had pedal edema and scotomata for several days. She had delivered a term infant in our hospital in 1960 and had no evidence at that time of hypertension nor of toxemia. She had had a poor protein intake during this pregnancy.

P.E.: Obese thirty-eight-year-old female in no distress. Blood pressure was 150/90. Estimated fetal weight was 3000 gms. There was a trace of pedal edema. Deep-tendon reflexes were normal.

Lab Data: Hematocrit: 33. Urine protein in twenty-four hours: negative. Serum uric acid: 6.7 mgm%. Serum urea nitrogen: 11 mgm%. Total serum proteins: 6.14 gm% with albumin

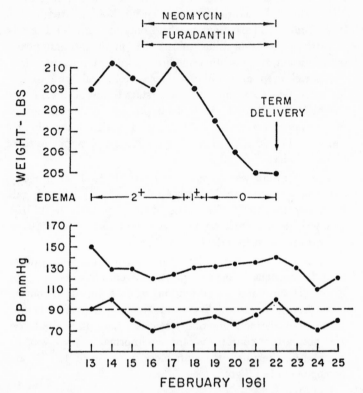

FIGURE 5. Mild toxemia. Patient lost 5 lbs in four days after starting neomycin; weight had been stable for five days. No salt restriction, no diuretic, full ambulation.

of 2.54 gm%. Quantitative urine culture was positive for E. coli in dilution greater than 100,000 organisms per ml.

Hospital Course (Fig. 5):

The patient was on a low salt diet and bed rest for forty-eight hours, during which time her weight remained stable between 209 and 210½ lbs. On the third hospital day, February 15, she was started on neomycin-sulfathalidine and furadantin (the latter for the symptomatic urinary tract infection which had developed). On the fifth day, February 17, she weighed 210¼ lbs and was started on a high protein diet. In the next four days she lost 5¼ lbs; her edema disappeared and her blood pressure remained normal. She had no diarrhea.

On February 22 she had the spontaneous rupture of her bag

of waters and began labor. Examination revealed a transverse lie, so she was delivered by means of Caesarean section of a 3272 gm female infant who did well. Her blood pressure was 140/100 for a few minutes while under anesthesia but remained normal otherwise and was 130-140/70-80 during the first eight hours postpartum and subsequently remained normal. The patient had no postpartum complications and was discharged on the seventh day with blood pressure of 110/70.

Case 4, D.R.

Hx: Twenty-year-old primigravida was admitted March 13, 1961 at twenty-four weeks gestation with prenatal care by a private physician for four visits. Her blood pressure had been normal in January, 1961. She had had headaches, scotomata and dizziness for several weeks. Weight gain by history was 15 lbs (109-124) and she had no edema. She had had a poor protein intake during this pregnancy.

P.E.: Apprehensive twenty-year-old female. Blood pressure was 160/110. Eyegrounds showed Grade I acute hypertensive changes. Estimated fetal weight was 1000 gm. There was no edema. Deep-tendon reflexes were slightly hyperactive.

Lab Data: Hematocrit: 41. Urine protein in 24 hours: 2.5 gm. Serum uric acid: 6.5 mgm%. Serum urea nitrogen: 13.0 mgm%. Total serum proteins: 5.50 gm% with 2.84 gm% albumin. Quantitative urine culture negative.

Hospital Course (Fig. 6):

The patient had mild, irregular, painful contractions throughout her hospital prenatal course. She was given neomycin-sulfathalidine on March 15; her blood pressure remained elevated for forty-eight hours and then fell to normal range. The fetal heart tones were last heard on March 18, and she stopped feeling movements of the fetus. She lost 8 lbs in five days. On March 20th she had four or five loose bowel movements. The neomycin-sulfa were discontinued March 20. Within four days she had gained back 4¾ lbs, and her blood pressure was 130/90 on March 21 and remained in the range of 120-130/80-90. On March 25 she delivered a macerated stillborn infant weighing 978 gm; there was a true knot pulled tight in the cord. Urine protein showed a steady decline, and there was only 4 mgm% in a random specimen the day prior to delivery. She had a normal postpartum course and was discharged on the third day.

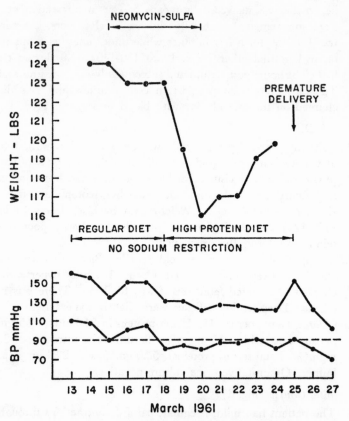

CASE NO. 4 D.R.

FIGURE 6. Twenty-year-old primigravida who had a poor protein intake during pregnancy. She had no edema but lost 8 lbs on neomycin-sulfathalidine; weight increased when antibiotics discontinued.

Case 5, B.L.

Hx: Twenty-four-year-old primigravida was admitted June 18, 1961, at thirty-six weeks gestation with no prenatal care. Two days prior to admission she had developed pain in the right flank and fever. By history she had gained 35 lbs (170-205) and had had edema of legs and ankles for several weeks. She had had scotomata for a week prior to admission with headaches. In 1956 at age nineteen she had a cholecystectomy and was told at that time that she had high blood pressure. She was unmarried, unhappily pregnant and had had a poor intake of protein during this pregnancy.

CASE NO. 5 B.L.

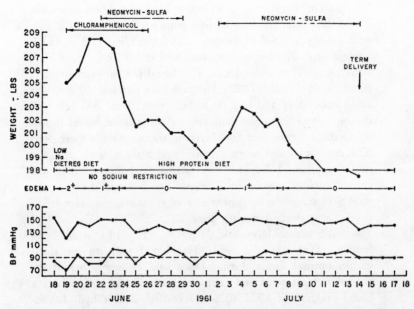

FIGURE 7. Twenty-four-year-old primigravida with poor protein intake during pregnancy. She was markedly obese with a past history of hypertension before she became pregnant; she had a urinary tract infection on admission. Patient lost 10½ lbs before delivery. Note reaccumulation of edema and weight gain when neomycin-sulfa discontinued. She had no diuretic and no sodium restriction after the first day and was fully ambulatory.

P.E.: Obese twenty-four-year-old female in moderate pain. Blood pressure 152/86. Eyegrounds showed acute hypertensive changes, Grade I. Estimated fetal weight was 3200 gm. There was moderate right costovertebral angle tenderness. Extremities showed two-plus pitting edema to the knees. Reflexes were normal.

Lab Data: Hematocrit: 36. Urine protein in twenty-four hours: 0.91 gram. Serum uric acid: 6.5 mgm%. Serum urea nitrogen: 7.0 mgm%. Total serum proteins: 6.0 gm% with 2.34 gm% albumin. Alk. phosphatase: 7.0 BU. Quantitative urine culture revealed E. coli greater than 100,000/ml. On June 24, six days after admission, a twenty-four-hour urinary excretion of urea nitrogen was 0.7 gm. On July 7, after two weeks on good protein diet, the twenty-four-hour excretion of urea nitrogen had risen to 4.8 gm.

Hospital Course (Fig. 7):

The patient was started on chloramphenicol for pyelonephritis. Three days later her weight had gone up from 205 to 208½, and she was started on neomycin-sulfathalidine and the high protein diet. She began a diuresis and lost 5 lbs in three days with disappearance of edema. Her blood pressure remained in the range 140-150/90-100. In nine days she lost 10 lbs, was fully ambulatory and had no sodium restriction. She felt well during this period. She had two or three loose bowel movements daily for the first five days and then one daily thereafter. The neomycin-sulfa were discontinued after a week and the patient gained 4 lbs and her edema reappeared. She was started back on neomycin-sulfa and lost 5 lbs in the next ten days with complete disappearance of edema again. Her urine protein was negligible after June 28.

She had a normal labor and delivery on July 14 of a 3374 gm female infant who did well. Her blood pressure remained within normal limits during labor and delivery; her deep-tendon reflexes remained normal. Immediately postpartum a blood pressure of 190/130 was recorded, and a hydralazine-cryptenamine drip was started. Blood pressure returned to 130/90 within twenty minutes, and the drip was stopped. Her blood pressure remained normal. She had a normal postpartum course and was discharged on the fourth postpartum day with blood pressure 140/80. (Her weight on the morning before delivery was 197½ lbs, 11 lbs less than the day the bowel antisepsis was started three weeks before.)

Case 6, G.D.

Hx: Twenty-four-year-old gravida 5 para 2 was admitted July 20, 1961, at thirty-six weeks gestation with no prenatal care. She came to the emergency room with the chief complaint that her feet were swollen and tight that it hurt her to walk. She had had generalized edema for three to four weeks with swelling of hands and face. Her weight gain by history was 73 lbs (170-243). She had had scotomata and headaches for several days prior to admission. She gave no history of hypertension nor of toxemia with her previous pregnancies. She had had a poor intake of protein during this pregnancy.

P.E.: Obese twenty-four-year-old female with generalized edema. Blood pressure was 170/100. Eyegrounds showed acute hypertensive changes, Grade I. Estimated fetal weight was 3400 gm. Extremities were markedly edematous; she was unable to make a fist because of edema of hands and fingers. There was

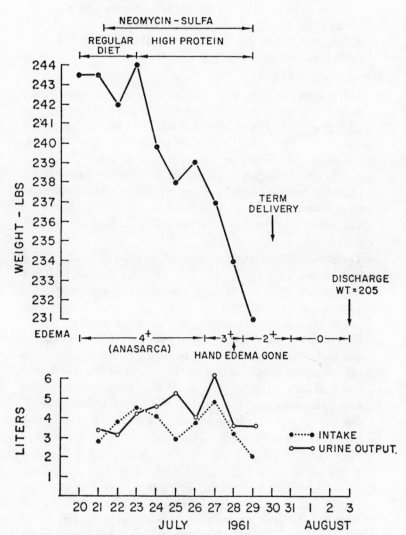

FIGURE 8. Markedly obese multipara with metabolic toxemia superimposed on chronic hypertension. She had massive edema on admission. Her protein intake during pregnancy had been very poor. She lost 13 lbs before delivery with no dietary salt restriction, no saluretic diuretic and full ambulation after the third hospital day.

four-plus edema extending over the lower abdominal wall. Deep-tendon reflexes were normal.

Lab Data: Hematocrit: 37. Urine protein in twenty-four hours: 0.40 gm. Serum uric acid: 6.7 mgm%. Serum urea nitrogen: 5.0 mgm%. Total serum proteins: 5.70 gm% with albumin of 2.39 gm%. Alk. phosphatase: 5.0 BU. Quantitative urine culture was negative.

Hospital Course (Fig. 8):

The patient was given 62.5 gm salt-poor serum albumin on the second hospital day and 25 gm on the third because of the massive edema; this produced a transient diuresis. She was started on neomycin-sulfathalidine in the evening of July 21, the second day. Her blood pressure went to 190/120, and she was given an intravenous drip of hydralazine-cryptenamine which dropped her blood pressure to 130/80. This resulted in an episode of anuria for three hours; when her blood pressure was allowed to return to the range 160/100, good urinary output ensued.

The blood pressure stabilized at 160-170/100-110, and her urine protein was 20 mgm%. On July 23, after forty-eight hours on neomycin-sulfa, she began a diuresis. The urine output on July 25 was over 5000 ml and there was appreciable decrease in her clinical edema. During this time she received phenobarbital 60 mgm every six hours; she was fully ambulatory and had no sodium restriction. In six days she lost thirteen lbs with complete disappearance of the edema of her hands and face and with marked improvement in lower extremity edema which diminished to two-plus at ankle level before delivery. On July 27, a week after admission, she put out 6200 ml urine with an intake of 4800 ml.

On July 29 at 2:00 A.M. she began to leak amniotic fluid and in the evening she had induction of labor with transbuccal pitocin and later augmented with intravenous drip of dilute pitocin. At 12:32 A.M. July 30, she had a normal spontaneous delivery of a 3260 gm male infant who did well. Her blood pressure went to 190/120 for a few minutes with a contraction in the second stage of labor and came down to 160/96 immediately postpartum and remained 160-170/90-100 until discharge on the fifth postpartum day at which time she weighed 205 lbs. She had an uneventful postpartum course.

Case 7, J.J.

Hx: Fourteen-year-old primigravida was admitted July 29, 1961, at thirty-five weeks gestation with no prenatal care. She came to the hospital because of marked swelling, burning and tightness of her feet and legs present for five to six weeks. She had had no headaches, scotomata nor other symptoms of toxemia. She had gained 14 lbs by history (121-135). She had a poor protein intake.

P.E.: Fourteen-year-old female with marked edema of lower extremities to knees and marked pallor of her mucus membranes. Blood pressure was 150/94. Eyegrounds were normal. Estimated fetal weight was 2500 gm. Extremities showed four-plus pitting edema to knees bilaterally. Deep-tendon reflexes were normal.

Lab Data: Hematocrit: 23. Urine protein in twenty-four hours:

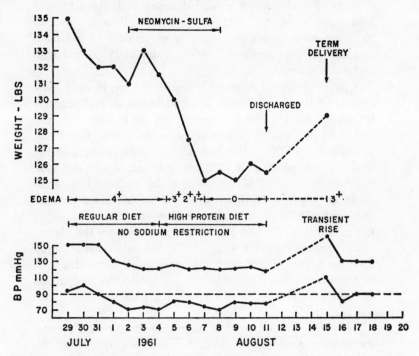

FIGURE 9. Fourteen-year-old primigravida with a history of poor protein intake during pregnancy. She lost 8 lbs on neomycin-sulfa with complete disappearance of edema which reaccumulated when antibiotics were discontinued. She had no saluretic diuretic, no dietary salt restriction and was fully ambulatory on the ward.

negative. Serum uric acid: 3.5 mgm%. Serum urea nitrogen: 6.0 mgm%. Alk. phosphatase: 5.3 BU. Sickle-cell prep: negative. Smear of peripheral blood: hypochromic, microcytic anemia, mean corpuscular volume 76. Quantitative urine culture was negative.

Hospital Course (Fig. 9):

The patient was observed for four days on a regular diet, and her weight dropped from 135 to 131, but the four-plus pitting edema of the lower extremities persisted. She was started on neomycin-sulfathalidine and subsequently on the high protein diet. The fifth day her weight had climbed back to 133, and then took a steady decline to 125 in the next four days, a loss of eight lbs. During this time her edema disappeared. Her blood pressure came down within normal limits before neomycin was begun and remained within normal limits until delivery. She developed a mild diarrhea with three to four loose stools daily. She was given ferrous sulfate for anemia. Neomycin-sulfa were discontinued after six days of treatment and she was discharged with weight stable at 125½ and with no trace of edema.

The patient returned August 15, four days later, in early labor and stated that her feet and legs had begun to swell the day before, August 14. She had gained 3½ lbs in four days and had three-plus pitting edema again to the knees. Her blood pressure was 130/90. She had an uneventful labor and delivery on August 16 of a 2835 gm male infant who did well. She had a transient hypertension under cyclopropane anesthesia to 180/110. However, during labor her blood pressure remained 130/80-90 and deep-tendon reflexes were always normal. During the first eight hours after delivery the highest blood pressure recorded was 132/80. She subsequently developed an acute urinary tract infection which responded well to antibiotics. She was discharged on the fourth postpartum day with normal blood pressure and no proteinuria.

Case 8, D.P.

Hx: This twenty-nine-year-old primigravida of estimated twenty-six weeks gestation was admitted to our hospital August 31, 1961, with the chief complaints of swelling of the legs for two months and swelling of the face and hands for two days. She had definite impairment of intelligence and could not recall her last menstrual period. She had seen a private physician for several visits, and had been on oral diuretics for a month. She had experienced nausea and anorexia for three days prior to admission. Her weight gain was estimated to be 30 lbs. She had a profuse vaginal discharge. Her protein intake had been poor.

P.E.: Markedly obese twenty-nine-year-old female with generalized edema. Blood pressure was 180/110. Weight 194½ lbs. Height 4 feet, 8 inches. Eyegrounds were normal. Extremities showed three-plus pedal, pre-tibial and hand edema with some facial edema. Deep-tendon reflexes were hyperactive.

Lab Data: Hematocrit: 32. Urine protein in twenty-four hours: 0.6 gm. Serum uric acid: 6.5 mgm%. Serum urea nitrogen: 5.0 mgm%. Total serum proteins: 5.90 gm% with albumin of 2.54 gm%. Alk. phosphatase: 4.1 BU. Quantitative urine culture revealed Pseudomonas greater than 100,000/ml.

Hospital Course (Fig. 10):

The patient was observed for two days on a regular diet and then bowel sterilization was begun; there was no sodium restriction. She received neomycin for eight days and tetracycline because of the positive urine culture. Her weight initially increased to 198 on August 3 and then began a steady drop to 181 on August 14 for a total loss of 17 lbs. During these eleven days she was fully ambulatory, ate her diet well and had complete disappearance of her edema. Her stools became loose on the third day. Her blood pressure remained in the range 130-150/80-90 except for one day on August 9 when it was recorded once at 180/100. She received no diuretic nor antihypertensive drugs. She received phenobarbital 30 mgm by mouth every six hours for four days. She had a monilial vaginitis treated with intravaginal jel, and the discharge improved.

The patient was discharged with careful dietary instructions August 15 and was subsequently seen as an outpatient August 22 and 29. On both these visits fetal heart tones were heard and her weight was stable at 181 lbs. She received chloramphenicol because of sensitivity studies of urine bacteria. She returned at 9:50 A.M., October 5, and was found to be fully dilated and effaced. She gave a history of a gush of fluid from her vagina at 2:30 A.M. of that day with onset of labor about that time. She was afebrile. Blood pressure was 150/100. Weight still 181 lbs. She had one-plus pre-tibial edema. She

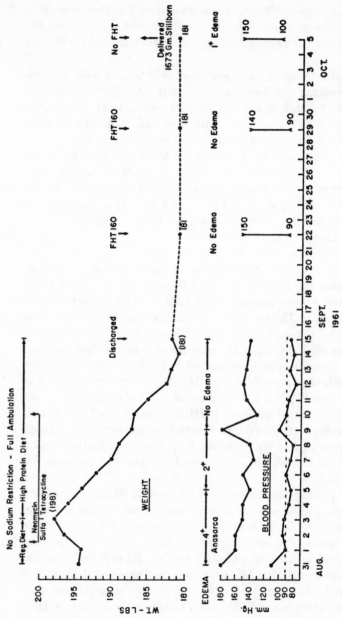
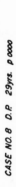

FIGURE 10. Markedly obese twenty-nine-year-old primigravida with a poor protein intake during pregnancy. Her height was 4 feet, 8 inches and her admission weight 194 lbs, which went to 198, and she then lost to 181 (18 lbs less) in twelve days. She had mild chronic hypertension with superimposed metabolic toxemia early in the third trimester. She had no diuretic, no dietary salt restriction and was fully ambulatory on the ward and at home. She delivered a congenitally deformed stillborn, but fetal heart tones were heard a week before delivery.

had a spontaneous delivery of a 1673 gm female stillborn infant at 10:21 A.M.; the infant showed signs of early maceration and had a congenitally deformed cervical vertebral column. The patient remained afebrile and had an uncomplicated postpartum course and was discharged on the second day with blood pressure of 150/90. A twenty-four-hour urine postpartum showed 0.6 gm protein.

Case 9, J.R.

Hx: Thirty-eight-year-old primigravida was admitted from our prenatal clinic on August 31, 1961, at thirty-six weeks gestation. She had had marked generalized edema for ten days and a total weight gain of 32 lbs. She had had nausea and vomiting for a week prior to admission and had headaches. She was unmarried, living with her elderly grandmother and quite emotionally stressed.

P.E.: A thirty-eight-year-old female with generalized edema. Blood pressure was 130/80. Weight 164 lbs. Eyegrounds were normal. Estimated fetal weight was 2500 gm. Extremities showed four-plus pitting edema of feet and legs and edema of fingers and hands. Deep-tendon reflexes were normal.

Lab Data: Hematocrit: 36. Urine protein in twenty-four hours: negative. Serum uric acid: 3.5 mgm%. Serum urea nitrogen: 7.0 mgm%. Total serum proteins: 4.60 gm% with albumin of 2.20 gm%. Rh negative; no antibodies demonstrated. Quantitative urine culture was negative.

Hospital Course (Fig. 11):

The patient was put on a low salt, high protein diet, bedrest, and was given 50 mgm hydrochlorothiazide by mouth four times daily for twelve doses. In four days she lost from 164 to 154½, 9½ lbs with complete disappearance of edema. On the fourth hospital day the diuretic was stopped, and she was started on a high protein diet with no sodium restriction and was encouraged to be ambulatory. She quickly regained the lost weight with reappearance of generalized edema; in seven days she gained 13½ lbs.

On September 9, neomycin-sulfathalidine were started. The patient remained edematous with weight stabilized at 168 for four days, then she began to mobilize edema fluid and lost 8 lbs in six days. Tetracycline was substituted for sulfathalidine on September 13. She developed a mild diarrhea on the fourth day which lasted three days.

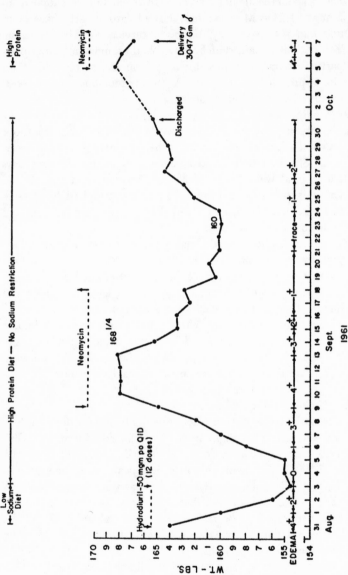
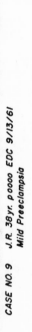

FIGURE 11. Thirty-eight-year-old emotionally disturbed primigravida with a history of a poor protein intake during pregnancy. She received excessive doses of a saluretic diuretic which produced a marked diuresis. Her edema reaccumulated rapidly when the diuretic was discontinued. She lost 8¾ lbs on neomycin and had a secondary reaccumulation of edema when it was discontinued.

There was a marked remission of edema, and by September 20 there was no clinical evidence of edema. She was fully ambulatory and ate well. Hypertension was never a significant problem with this patient, and only on a few occasions near her delivery was a pressure of 160/90 recorded.

On September 18 the neomycin was discontinued and tetracycline was stopped three days later. On September 24, six days after stopping neomycin, the patient began to develop edema again; in three days she gained 4½ lbs and developed two-plus pedal and pre-tibial edema. Because of emotional problems she was discharged on October 1 at which time she weighed 165 and had two-plus lower extremity edema.

The patient was readmitted on October 5 and had gained 3½ more lbs in five days with considerable increase in edema of her lower extremities. Blood pressure was 150/90. She was started back on neomycin and showed some regression of edema before her spontaneous delivery at 1:43 A.M., October 8 of a 3042 gm male infant who did well. She developed a vulvar hematoma which was evacuated and a bleeding vessel found and sutured in the episiotomy wound.

The patient had an uneventful postpartum course and was discharged on the sixth day with a blood pressure of 130/70. She returned for a six weeks' check and was normotensive and doing well.

Case 10, H.P.

Hx: Twenty-six-year-old primigravida admitted January 29, 1962, at thirty-five weeks gestation because of marked edema of the lower extremities for one month and hypertension. She had made eight prenatal visits to the county clinic. At each visit she had complained about constant nausea and vomiting but nothing was done to correct it. She consequently had a very poor diet during this pregnancy and a low protein intake. Her weight gain was twenty-six lbs (82-108). An x-ray on Dec. 1 had demonstrated a twin gestation. She had had an upper respiratory infection for a week and for two days a Bell's palsy. Her blood pressure had been normal until the last clinic visit and she had had no previous proteinuria.

P.E.: Poorly nourished, emaciated twenty-six-year-old female with a left peripheral facial palsy. Blood pressure was 150/100. Estimated fetal weight was 1800 gm for each twin. There

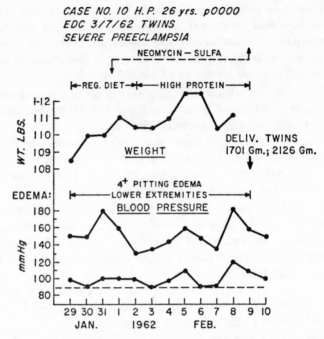

FIGURE 12. Severe metabolic toxemia of late pregnancy in a twenty-six-year-old primigravida with twins. She had a very poor intake of protein during pregnancy and had vomited continuously throughout. She showed no response to intestinal sterilization and high protein diet; she was unable to take diet well. This patient had "liver palms."

was three-plus pitting edema to the knees. Deep-tendon reflexes were hyperactive. Patient had "liver palms."

Lab Data: Hematocrit: 35. Urine protein in twenty-four hours: 2.0 gm. Serum uric acid: 6.1 mgm%. Serum urea nitrogen: 12.0 mgm%. Total serum proteins: 6.60 gm% with albumin 2.18 gm%. Alk. Phosphatase: 18.1 BU (when the alkaline phosphatase was repeated seven days later it was 16.4 BU.) Cephalin flocculation was one-plus.

Hospital Course (Fig. 12):

The patient was put on neomycin-sulfathalidine, Vit. K, phenobarbital and a high protein diet which she ate poorly. In nine days of therapy there was no response in her blood pressure which remained 140-160/90-120. Her weight increased from 108½ to 111 on the day of delivery. After five days her appetite began to improve somewhat but was never good. She continued to spill about 100 mgm% protein in the urine. There was no diminution of peripheral edema. She developed diarrhea on the second day of therapy.

On February 9 at 9:00 P.M. there was a spontaneous rupture of the amniotic sac of one twin and the patient went into labor. Her blood pressure went up to 180/120, and she was given an antihypertensive drip. She delivered twins after nine hours of labor; they weighed 1701 gm and 2126 gm and did well. The patient had normal blood pressure and no proteinuria by the fifth postpartum day.

"Control" Patients

Three patients with evidence of mild toxemia were studied and managed in a manner similar to those above except they were not given neomycin and sulfathalidine. They received a high protein diet with no sodium restriction after therapy was established, were fully ambulatory and received a minimum of symptomatic drugs.

Case 11, M.V.

Hx: Twenty-one-year-old primigravida of thirty-five weeks gestation was admitted to our labor unit from the prenatal clinic November 6, 1961, because of blood pressure of 145/90, edema and hyperactive reflexes. She had had headaches and dizziness for two weeks and a history of a forty-one-lb weight gain. She had made one previous prenatal visit on October 26 at which time her blood pressure was 136/80 and there was no edema and no proteinuria. She had had a poor protein intake during pregnancy.

P.E.: Twenty-one-year-old female in no distress with mild edema. Blood pressure was 140/90. Weight 153 lbs. Eyegrounds showed Grade I acute hypertensive changes. Estimated fetal weight was 3000 gm. Lower extremities showed one-plus edema with slight edema of hands. Deep-tendon reflexes were hyperactive.

Lab Data: Hematocrit: 33. Urine protein in twenty-four hours: negative. Serum uric acid: 6.1 mgm%. Serum urea nitrogen: 11.0 mgm%. Total serum proteins: 6.00 gm% with albumin of 3.04 gms%. Rh negative; no antibodies. Quantitative urine culture revealed a gamma streptococcus greater than 100,000/ml, heat resistant, coagulase negative.

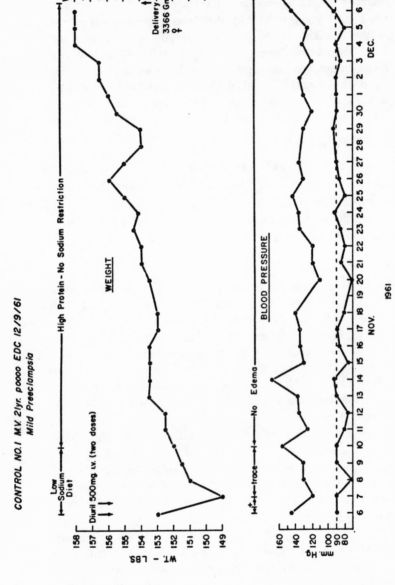

FIGURE 13. Mild metabolic toxemia of late pregnancy in a twenty-one-year-old primigravida who had a poor intake of protein during pregnancy. She had no weight loss after initial 4-lb loss on diuretic. Clinical edema did not re-accumulate; she gained 9 lbs before delivery. (Compare with Fig. 7.)

Hospital Course (Fig. 13):

The patient was given 500 mgm chlorothiazide intravenously on November 6, the day of admission, and a similar dose the next day and then no further diuretics. She was started on a high protein diet with low salt and bed rest. She lost from 153 to 149½ in a twenty-four-hour period. On November 10 she was started on a high protein diet with no sodium restriction and was encouraged to ambulate freely. She gradually gained over a four-week period to 158 on the day prior to delivery. Her urine remained negative for protein throughout and she had no clinical edema after November 10. Her diastolic pressure remained in the vicinity of 90 mm until she went into labor. On December 6 at 3:15 P.M. the membranes ruptured spontaneously and she developed irregular contractions. A pitocin stimulation with dilute intravenous drip was given; her blood pressure went up to 160/110. She had an otherwise normal labor and delivery at 2:18 P.M. on December 7 of a 3366 gm female infant who did well. She had a normal postpartum course and was discharged on the fifth day with blood pressure of 120/70.

Case 12, C.C.

Hx: Thirty-three-year-old primigravida of thirty-seven weeks gestation was admitted November 15, 1961, at her first prenatal clinic visit because of generalized edema and a blood pressure of 150/100. For six weeks she had edema of the lower extremities and for three days she had noticed swelling of her hands and blurring of vision. She had had headaches and dizziness for about three weeks. She had a poor protein intake during pregnancy. Her weight gain by history was 30 lbs.

P.E.: Thirty-three-year-old female in no acute distress. Blood pressure was 150/100. Eyegrounds showed Grade I acute hypertensive changes. Estimated fetal weight was 2600 gm. There was three-plus edema of lower extremities and hands. Deep-tendon reflexes were normal.

Lab Data: Hematocrit: 33. Urine protein in twenty-four hours: 0.64 gm. Serum uric acid: 8.1 mgm%. Serum urea nitrogen: 12.0 mgm%. Quantitative urine culture revealed a micrococcus greater than 100,000/ml, coagulase negative.

Hospital Course (Fig. 14):

The patient was initially treated with bed rest, low salt, high protein diet, and she was given hydrochlorothiazide 50 mgm by mouth every eight hours for four doses, phenobarbital 30

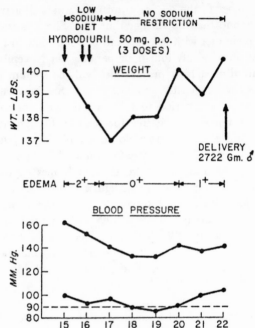

FIGURE 14. Thirty-three-year-old primigravida with mild metabolic toxemia. She gave a history of inadequate protein intake during pregnancy. She had no weight loss after initial response to diuretic; there was reaccumulation of edema fluid before delivery.

mgm p.o. q six hours for seven doses and hydralazine 24 mgm p.o. q four hours for five doses. These medications were then discontinued on November 17. She lost 3 lbs the first two days and gained it back in three days. Her blood pressure remained in the vicinity of 140/90. On November 20 she was started on tetracycline because of the positive urine culture. She delivered uneventfully at 8:15 A.M. on November 22 a 2722 gm male infant who did well. Her weight was 140½ on the morning of delivery, one half pound more than on admission a week before. Her postpartum course was normal and she was discharged on the fourth day with blood pressure of 130/90.

Case 13, H.R.

Hx: Thirty-five-year-old mentally retarded gravida 4 para 1 was admitted November 16, 1961, because of scotomata and marked edema of lower extremities. She was of estimated thirty-eight weeks gestation. Her weight gain was not known. She had been living in a nursing home of some sort but no history was available.

P.E.: Thirty-five-year-old mentally retarded female; blood pressure was 110/70. Eyegrounds were normal. Estimated fetal weight was 3400 gm. There was marked edema of the lower extremities including thighs. Deep-tendon reflexes were normal.

Lab Data: Hematocrit: 39. Urine protein in twenty-four hours: negative. Serum uric acid: 4.0 mgm%. Serum urea nitrogen: 6.0 mgm%. Total serum proteins: 5.70 gm% with albumin of 2.16 gm%. Alk. phosphatase 9.6 BU. Quantitative urine culture was negative.

Hospital Course (Fig. 15):

The patient was treated with a high protein diet with no sodium restriction and no diuretics. She gained initially from 136½ to 139 and then lost to 135 in four days, and her weight re-

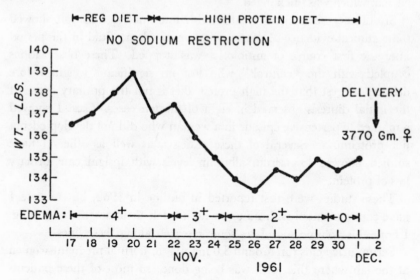

FIGURE 15. Clinical edema subsided on high protein diet but there was no significant weight loss before delivery.

mained stable at 135 lbs until delivery. Her blood pressure remained normal until she began labor, when it went to 140/88 and was 154/100 immediately postpartum, and it returned to normal four hours after delivery. She had a normal labor and a spontaneous delivery at 7:00 P.M., December 2 of a 3696 gm infant who did well. The patient had a normal postpartum course.

Comments

I do not report these studies as clinical therapeutic trials, but rather I wanted to test the concept that hepatic detoxication systems might be relieved of a load of aromatic compounds arising from the lower GI tract. I believe the clinical data support this concept. Case 10 represents a severely malnourished woman with twins. Her clinical toxemia was most severe, and I would not expect to be able to treat her very effectively except by delivering her. Her protein reserves are very low. After delivery and mobilization of her edema fluid she weighed only 72 lbs (height about 5 ft, 2 in) and looked as if she had just come out of a concentration camp. The fact that she had a mild diarrhea did not cause her to lose weight nor to mobilize her edema, which was unchanged.

Six of the ten patients treated with intestinal sterilization showed some clinical evidence of *reaccumulation* of edema fluid in the period after the first course of antibiotics was stopped. These observations coupled with the "controls" who lost no significant weight before delivery suggest that the high protein diet is not the primary cause of the initial diuresis observed in eight of the ten cases. Case 1 showed a marked hypertensive episode in a woman who did not develop edema nor proteinuria. Several of these patients, as well as others I have studied, showed low serum albumin levels with insignificant urinary loss of protein.

These studies were first reported in outline in 1962, but to date I have communicated with no one who has felt them worth confirming. I hope this volume stimulates some research along these lines.

Serum uric acids run around 3.0 mgm% in normal pregnant women at the lab where this work was being done; so most of these patients had definitely elevated serum uric acid levels. The variations in clinical manifestations of MTLP may well be related to the specific strains of bacteria present in the GI tract as well as to the specific deficiencies of nutritional elements which may be quite complex. It is clear that sodium retention and hypertension usually precede more severe tissue damage as revealed in proteinuria and more profound abnormalities in hepatic function.

I followed each one of these patients carefully and made a real effort to see that they ate their diets well and stayed out of bed as much as possible. Also I included a salt shaker on their trays and encouraged them to salt their food to taste. We have all observed marked diureses in patients with mild toxemia just from putting them at bed rest and giving them a hospital diet. I also tried to make as careful differential diagnosis as possible—as outlined in Chapter 2—and consequently turned down a number of patients admitted by other residents as "toxemia" but who on study turned out to have some other similar clinical disorder.

TOXIC ABRUPTIO PLACENTAE

Premature separation of a normally implanted placenta often occurs in our southern states among women in our lowest socioeconomic class associated with severe MTLP. I will refer to this as "toxic abruptio placentae," for I consider it one of the severe manifestations of the underlying metabolic disease. I think it is directly analogous to the abruptions of the placenta which McKay has produced by feeding pregnant rats a low protein, high oxidized fat diet. Hibbard of Liverpool has recently reported evidence that abruptio placentae in his area is associated with folic acid deficiency. He did not note a high correlation with MTLP, and this suggests that the woman who develops MTLP in our southern states associated with abruptio has multiple dietary deficiencies and/or the specific bacterial flora in her GI tract may be particularly biochemically malignant, that is, certain strains of bacteria may produce more potentially toxic compounds than others and thereby make greater demands on the liver and damage it more easily. There is strong evidence that good nutrition will prevent this toxic abruption of the placenta. Recently I talked with an obstetrician who has practiced here in the San Francisco Bay Area for over twenty years and has not had one of his private patients develop this sometimes lethal complication. It is possible to see two or three such cases come in during a thirty-six-hour shift working in our big city-county hospital labor units in the South.

It is a clinical teaching passed from resident to resident in our southern hospitals that when you first encounter a patient with a toxic abruption, you are "already three units (1500 ml) of blood behind." These women undoubtedly have markedly contracted blood volumes *before* they have the abruption and begin to bleed, either externally or behind the placenta. This contracted blood volume plays a role in the pathogenesis of the abruption. It has long been observed clinically that these women develop signs of blood-loss shock "out of proportion" to the amount of blood lost. These women occasionally develop anuria associated with renal cortical or tubular necrosis, and this must be caused by a prolonged period of inadequate renal blood flow. For these reasons it is necessary to be liberal in transfusing these women and to avoid procrastination in getting them delivered if their lives are to be saved. The use of intravenous human serum albumin to expand plasma volume and to improve renal plasma flow in these women needs to be investigated.

During four years of residency at Jackson Memorial Hospital, where I helped care for a number of severely ill women with toxic abruptio placentae, certain ideas occurred to me concerning the pathogenesis of this serious complication. What are the common biochemical and physiological conditions associated with MTLP which could lead to the premature separation of a normally implanted placenta? Elizabeth Ramsey and her co-workers have given us a clear, scientific picture of how the placental circulation works. Maternal blood enters the intervillous space from the endometrial spiral arterioles in discrete, relatively high pressure funnel-shaped streams or jets. Blood is drained from the intervillous space by small uterine veins on the floor of the intervillous space. Thus, the placenta has been shown anatomically to be an arteriovenous shunt, a condition for which we have had good evidence from clinical physiological observations.[38] Any conditions which will lead to clot formation in the intervillous space may be regarded as playing some role in the pathogenesis of abruption.

The following factors occur in severe MTLP and can play a role in promoting the formation of a clot behind the placenta:

1. Reduction in velocity of blood flowing through the intervillous

space associated with arteriolar spasm (of uterine spiral arterioles);

2. Increased viscosity of maternal blood associated with hemoconcentration, hypoalbuminemia and hypovolemia;

3. Increased fibrinogen concentration of maternal blood associated with hemoconcentration and probably hepatic injury; and

4. Widespread endothelial injury of unknown cause which can damage the fetal cotyledons and release thromboplastin to trigger the clotting mechanism.

Much clinical interest has been focused on hypofibrinogenemia in abruptio placentae, but it develops in a relatively small percentage of cases. I agree with Pritchard that this hypofibrinogenemia is related to loss of fibrin from the blood. In some women the liver is unable to synthesize fibrinogen fast enough to keep up with the loss. Hypofibrinogenemia has recently been reported in a variety of bleeding complications of pregnancy including placenta praevia, abortion, ruptured ectopic pregnancy and postpartum hemorrhage. Further research will elucidate this question.

It is of much practical clinical importance for the obstetrician to view toxic abruptio placentae as one of the manifestations of an underlying *metabolic disease,* for then it will emphasize in his mind the vital importance of a careful differential diagnosis of third trimester hemorrhage. The basic differences between the mechanical separation of the marginal sinus, as the cervix begins to efface and dilate and a toxic abruption associated with profound physiological and biochemical abnormalities will indicate the greatly increased hazards to both mother and infant in the latter case. It will be understood why it is a definite mistake to classify bleeding from a ruptured marginal sinus, which is a mechanical problem, as a "first degree abruption." This indicates that it might progress into a "second degree" or "third degree" abruption. Likewise, *any degree* of abruption associated with MTLP will be seen clearly as an immediate hazard to fetal survival, for the placenta may abrupt totally at any time when conditions develop as outlined above. Among our improverished and malnourished women in the southern states with severe toxic abruptio placentae, approximately 50 per cent have already had intrauterine fetal deaths before they reach the labor unit. An alert resident staff is often responsible for saving the life of an infant when fetal heart tones are heard on admission and a rapid delivery can be effected. When fetal heart tones are not heard on admission, immediate delivery is likewise indicated to minimize maternal blood loss, shock and damage to the maternal kidneys which can lead to death.

RENAL DYSFUNCTION

A review of the medical literature on this subject of renal function in toxemia of pregnancy would make up a large volume. I think renal dysfunction is of *secondary significance* in metabolic toxemia of late pregnancy. As an obstetrical resident at Jackson Memorial Hospital, I could never get the renal physiologists very interested in our usual toxemic patients. "If her BUN is normal, get her delivered and her kidneys will be all right" is the answer I used to get in requests for consultation. I wanted to learn something from them about this peculiar "kidney disease" of pregnancy in which the serum urea nitrogen levels were always normal or low in spite of a glomerular lesion. I suspected that the reduction in glomerular filtration rate which was discussed so widely in the literature was only secondary to a primary reduction in renal plasma flow. I finally resolved this problem in my mind by clinical observations made on women following delivery which often causes immediate and dramatic increases in urinary output in oliguric toxemic women. Infusions of human serum albumin, I learned from experience, will also produce dramatic diureses in the sickest patients before delivery.

How then can the toxemic glomerular lesion so extensively studied by both light and electron microscope be of much physiological significance when increasing the renal blood flow results in diureses? It is obvious that in the great majority of women with MTLP renal dysfunction it not a significant problem. Of course if the diagnosis is not correct, and the woman really has an underlying renal disease with or without MTLP, then the situation is different. Also it has been emphasized how the maternal kidneys can be damaged by shock as in abruptio placentae with hemorrhage.

The injudicious use of saluretic diuretics which further shrink a contracted blood volume and reduce renal plasma flow may bring on profound renal dysfunction. The serum urea nitrogen may rise over

100 mgm% as the patient, often kept on a very low sodium intake, develops the "low salt syndrome." Even these patients will usually improve dramatically if the situation is correctly diagnosed and salt added to their diets and the diuretics stopped immediately. Profound potassium depletion may also occur in pregnant women treated with saluretic diuretics.

Table II demonstrates some of the striking differences between severe MTLP and glomerulonephritis, with which it is often compared in the clinician's mind because of the superficial similarity of the two diseases.

TABLE II

COMPARISON OF SOME OF THE PHYSIOLOGICAL MANIFESTA-
TIONS OF ACUTE GLOMERULONEPHRITIS, A PRIMARY RENAL
DISEASE INVOLVING THE GLOMERULUS OF THE RENAL
NEPHRON, WITH SEVERE METABOLIC TOXEMIA OF LATE
PREGNANCY WHICH IS NOT A PRIMARY RENAL DISEASE

Acute Glomerulonephritis	*Severe Metabolic Toxemia of Late Pregnancy*
1. Plasma volume normal or increased	1. Plasma volume reduced
2. Hemodilution	2. Hemoconcentration
3. Serum proteins normal	3. Serum proteins reduced, especially low albumin
4. Serum urea nitrogen and creatinine elevated	4. Serum urea nitrogen and creatinine normal or low
5. Serum uric acid elevated in proportion to urea nitrogen elevation	5. Serum uric acid often elevated with low serum urea nitrogen
6. Proteinuria constant from day to day; often over 5.0 gm in 24 hours	6. Proteinuria fluctuates; seldom over 5.0 gm in 24 hours
7. Casts, cells prominent in urine	7. Few casts or cells in urine except in terminal oliguria
8. Hypertension constant from hour to hour and from day to day	8. Hypertension fluctuates from hour to hour and day to day, labile

CENTRAL NERVOUS SYSTEM DYSFUNCTION

The severely toxemic woman may be disoriented in time and space before or after convulsions which are generalized, of the grand mal type. She may lapse into coma without having convulsions. Her deep-tendon reflexes are often hyperactive preceding convulsions, but equally hyperactive reflexes may be found in excitable women in labor or before without any underlying problem of MTLP. Headache is a prominent symptom in MTLP. Women with MTLP may develop an associated cerebrovascular accident in which the neurological signs and symptoms will be determined by the site and extent of the lesion. In many hospitals in our nation, convulsions due to MTLP make up a definite minority of cases of convulsions occuring in pregnant women.

I do not know the cause of these eclamptic convulsions. I look on the coma as being that of a severe terminal hepatic disease.

HOW DELIVERY OF THE PLACENTA AND FETUS IMPROVES THE CLINICAL CONDITION OF THE TOXEMIC PATIENT

Now that we have acquired some understanding of the basic biochemical and physiological abnormalities associated with this disease process, we can grasp the basic factors which result in improvement following delivery of the placenta and fetus.

1. The arteriovenous shunt effect of the placenta is removed; the uterus contracts and reduces uterine blood flow markedly so that this blood is now available for renal perfusion.
2. The placental source of steroid hormones is removed so the liver cells are immediately relieved of the metabolic burden of detoxifying them. Progesterone may disappear from the blood within five minutes after delivery. Hepatic detoxication of other aromatic potentially toxic compounds may thus be more effective.
3. The nutritional burden of the fetus is removed.
4. The patient's appetite may improve, leading to improved nutrition.
5. The gastrointestinal tract is no longer compressed and crowded.

It is an old assumption firmly rooted in clinical thinking that intrauterine fetal death is always associated with improvement in the clinical condition of the toxemic patient. This has not been my experience, and looking over the literature, I find that others have cast doubt on the validity of this assumption. Dexter and Weiss, in a study on the effect of intrauterine fetal death on maternal blood pressure and proteinuria of sixteen patients with toxemia of pregnancy, found:

1. No clinical improvement in eleven patients;
2. Partial or complete improvement in five patients;
3. In two cases, generalized edema became more profound after intrauterine fetal death.

These observations suggested to Weiss and Dexter that improvement in toxemia occuring after delivery was caused primarily due to removal of the placenta and not the fetus.

CHAPTER 5

ETIOLOGY

W<small>ITH A CLEAR AND DEFINITE</small> conception of metabolic toxemia of late pregnancy as a clinical disease entity, with an understanding of the importance of its complex differential diagnosis, with some basic knowledge of its abnormal physiology and biochemistry, we are in a better position to understand its basic *cause.*

Hans Selye wrote in 1955:

> . . . the main objects of our researches are no longer individual pathogens but rather *pathogenic situations.*

We come to study phenomena as being interrelated in complex chains of events; we study and attempt to describe *conditions* which result in abnormal patterns of physiology and biochemistry in diseases. In this broad sense, metabolic toxemia of late pregnancy is *caused* by any conditions, socioeconomic, physiologic, biochemical or psychological, which result in *malnutrition.* The pregnant woman who develops this disease has failed to get into her *internal milieu,* into her general metabolism, all the essential elements of nutrition in the correct amounts and proportions to meet the increased nutritional demands of her own particular pregnancy.

From this point of view we can understand immediately how both multiple pregnancy and diabetes mellitus can alter the nutritional requirements, both qualitatively and quantitatively, increasing them above the nutritional requirements of a nondiabetic woman with a single fetus. We can understand how the nutritional status, including her dietary habits, of a woman before she becomes pregnant is important in determining her pregnancy outcome. We can also confidently predict that every pregnant woman who is able to eat, digest, absorb, and metabolize normally an adequate diet for her pregnancy will not develop metabolic toxemia of late pregnancy. This implies normal liver function.

This basic knowledge about MTLP will enable the clinician to practically eradicate the disease among all women who come to him early in pregnancy for prenatal care. It will cause him to question and to avoid all current clinical practices which in any way interfere with good, well-balanced nutrition throughout pregnancy. It will cause him to treat aggressively any conditions which threaten to interfere with good prenatal nutrition. It will be of considerable aid in the differential diagnosis in any woman who develops hypertension, edema, proteinuria, convulsions, coma and other signs of "toxemia."

Of the fact that malnutrition causes fundamental changes in metabolism of hepatic cells during pregnancy, there is no doubt. The clinical manifestations of MTLP vary greatly from patient to patient, and this is undoubtedly due to the complexity of nutritional deficiencies, variations in production of placental hormones by the placenta and to variations in bacterial flora of the gastrointestinal tract. A great deal more basic knowledge about this disease process can be acquired. The exact biochemical nature of the malnutrition is unknown; evidence is strong that essential amino acids, contained in high biological quality proteins, may be deficient in the diets of women who develop MTLP. An associated high fat intake may play a significant role. The biochemical causes of the endothelial lesions found widely about the body in this disease process are unknown. These questions are briefly discussed in the last chapter.

This book is presented at this time because enough reliable scientific knowledge is available about metabolic toxemia of late pregnancy to accurately diagnose it, to treat it rationally and not blindly aim at its symptoms, and, most important of all, *to prevent it.* The clear conception that metabolic toxemia of late pregnancy is a disease of *nutritional deficiency* mediated through *hepatic dysfunction* should speed acquisition of more basic biochemical knowledge.

CHAPTER 6

OBESITY, WEIGHT GAIN, DIETARY SALT AND DIURETICS: A PERSPECTIVE

OBESITY

OBESITY IS OFTEN thought of as being a form of "malnutrition," and in a certain sense it is. However, it is necessary for the clinician to recognize that an obese woman may be perfectly well nourished from the point of view of her taking in all the necessary elements of nutrition. She may get fat from eating too much of a biologically adequate diet. I had occasion to make a house call to see a young child with middle-ear infection during my general practice days. His mother, a very obese woman of short stature (weight 195 lbs, height 4 ft, 10 in), related to me her prenatal experiences. She had delivered three infants, and during each pregnancy she maintained her marked obesity; her obstetrician was apprehensive about her developing toxemia with each, but she had no trouble at all with any of her pregnancies. How did you eat during your pregnancies?" I asked her.

"Oh, I ate like a horse; I especially like meat and milk." This woman's husband is a civil engineer with a good position and salary, and she was "kitchen oriented," that is, she delighted in preparing good food and enjoyed eating it.

On the other side of the coin we know that many obese women are very poorly nourished because they eat too much carbohydrate and fat and very little protein. I helped care for a young woman who ate like this and died of eclampsia. It is not possible to distinguish from casual observation the adequately nourished obese woman from the poorly nourished one, and therefore it is necessary to take a careful dietary history and to do certain lab studies to clarify the situation. Studies done on obese women in private practice in this nation have shown that obesity, *per se,* does not predispose a woman to developing serious maternal complications, while studies done on obese women

[69]

in the lower socioeconomic classes have revealed an increased incidence of such complications.[40, 41]

In the management of the obese pregnant woman, physicians often make one serious mistake: they restrict dietary intake so much that protein deficiency develops. I have observed this phenomenon in ten women who thus developed "iatrogenic" metabolic toxemia of late pregnancy. (Controlled experimental studies done on lower primates will reveal the same phenomenon.) One of the most striking cases occurred in a woman twenty-eight years of age having her first pregnancy. I saw her first two days after her admission to the obstetrical prenatal ward of a university hospital. She had been referred into the hospital by her private physician, who had been looking after her since the first trimester. She was twenty-eight weeks gestation on admission. She was a college graduate, an intelligent and cooperative woman. On admission she had hypertension, proteinuria, generalized edema and was having symptoms of MTLP. She had been placed on a low salt diet and a saluretic diuretic, sedation, bed rest and the other "routine therapy" for "toxemia of pregnancy." A very poor history was on her chart.

As I elicited a fairly detailed history, it became obvious what her problem was and how it had developed. Early in pregnancy she was somewhat overweight, being 5 feet, 7 inches tall and weighing about 175 lbs. Her physician placed her on a starvation diet of 400 cal and strengthened her will to fight her good appetite with amphetamines. She faithfully followed this diet, but in spite of it, as pregnancy advanced into the latter half she continued to gain weight. Six weeks prior to admission, she developed clinical edema so the physician placed her on oral saluretic diuretics and advised salt restriction and continued her on the 400-cal diet. She followed this regimen faithfully also but continued to develop progressively severe signs and symptoms of MTLP, including proteinuria. Her physician then referred her into the university hospital for more expert care.

It is obvious that the obstetrical resident's initial plan of therapy was unscientific because of his failure to take an adequate history and to find out as much as possible about the events which preceded the patient's admission to the hospital. The diuretic was stopped. A serum sodium revealed a concentration of 118 me/liter; a total serum protein was 5.4 gm% with albumin of 1.80 gm% (by electro-phoresis). The patient was given sodium and taken off the low sodium diet. After ten days during which she showed slight improve-ment, she went into labor spontaneously and delivered a 2100 gm premature infant which suffered the respiratory distress syndrome but survived. (It is of interest to note that the total serum proteins on the infant's cord blood were only 4.8 gm%, and it was given some intravenous human serum albumin.)

On the day of the patient's discharge from the hospital I talked with her husband to verify her history. He was quite perplexed as he told me: "I just don't understand it; she followed the doctor's orders to the letter. She starved herself throughout this pregnancy eating less in a day than she used to eat in one meal, and yet she continued to gain weight and got sick."

It is perfectly safe for obese women to diet during pregnancy pro-vided they have an adequate intake of protein and of all the essential elements of good nutrition. However, it is much more important for the obese woman to eat a good adequate diet than it is for her to lose weight during pregnancy. It is necessary for the physician and his patient to place the primary interest on good nutrition, since the obese woman may have poor dietary habits; weight reduction must be looked on as a secondary and less important goal.

Weight Gain

Nowhere in medicine are statistics more abused than in modern obstetrics. The information learned from studying a thousand cases from hospital records can not replace a detailed clinical study of the individual patient. False conclusions drawn from many statistical studies about weight gain in pregnancy have clouded understanding and rational practice for many years.

It is clear that a sudden rapid weight gain may be one of the first manifestations of toxemia of late pregnancy. However, we often see severe toxemia in women who failed to gain enough. Among indigent women in the southern states, failure to gain ten pounds or more dur-ing pregnancy is an indication of poor nutrition and a significant num-ber of women in this group develop MTLP. We have also observed women who gained forty or fifty pounds during pregnancy and had normal prenatal courses and produced healthy infants. These observations seem confusing until one grasps the basic concept that an obese woman may be "well nourished."

There are thus two distinct categories for excessive weight gain;

1. Excess tissue deposits, chiefly of fat but some protein is stored; and
2. Excess fluid retention.

Both mechanisms may operate in the same woman. Women in the first category may be quite adequately nourished or very poorly nourished depending on their individual experiences. Again we see the importance of taking a thorough clinical history in order to understand the individual patient.

The misplaced emphasis placed on "weight gain" by many modern obstetricians leads to some undesirable consequences. Many women have told me that their physician made such a fuss over their weight gain that they were afraid to go in for the prenatal visit. Women often starve themselves for several days prior to the prenatal appointment, particularly if they have gained excessively. Many women take castor oil or some other strong cathartic the day before the prenatal visit. Women become so preoccupied with keeping their weight down that they fail to place proper emphasis on the principles of good nutrition. Many women with common sense continue to eat a good diet in the face of their physician's criticisms and disapproval, and this leads to a certain discord and disrupts the patient-physician relationship which is important in the psychological preparation of the patient for labor and delivery. All these vexing situations can be eliminated when physician and patient grasp the basic ideas presented here.

DIETARY SALT AND DIURETICS

My own clinical experiences working with many normal and toxemic pregnant women have led me to the firm conviction that restriction of salt in the diet of pregnant women produces no clinical benefit. Several investigators in this country and in England and Canada have recorded similar experiences.[43, 44, 45] Of course this does not apply to the woman with significant cardiovascular or renal disease during pregnancy.

Salt restriction has some undesirable results, particularly when combined with the use of saluretic diuretics. Many women have told me that both physicians and public health nurses had told them not to drink milk because it contains too much salt. This is wrong, because milk is one of the most important and cheapest sources we have available for high biological quality proteins. A low salt diet is not very savory, and the patients often do not eat well when actually following such a diet.

It is in the hospitalized patients that one of the most glaring errors is often made in pregnancy nutrition. Here we have opportunity to provide the patient with an optimum diet planned and prepared by expert nutritionists. I have been in several hospitals in our nation where the routine management of the toxemic patient calls for a "low salt diet" which on inquiry is found to contain only 50 gm of protein. To reduce the toxemic patient's protein intake below that of the requirements of normal pregnancy is to make a grave physiological and biochemical mistake.

Figure 11 (Chap. 4, p. 52) demonstrates a common clinical phenomenon: a diuretic which causes the kidneys to excrete an excessive amount of sodium and potassium, and water associated therewith does not have any effect upon the underlying metabolic disorder in MTLP, for as soon as the diuretic is stopped, the sodium and water retention immediately recurs. A diuresis may blind the physician to the fact that the patient is really getting worse. Diuretics are absolutely contraindicated in the severely toxemic patient who has a contracted blood volume, low serum albumin and hemoconcentration. The following three cases are presented in detail to illustrate the clinical reality of these ideas. It was from the careful study of these and other similar cases that I began to crystallize my ideas about the pathogenesis of metabolic toxemia of late pregnancy and to turn from concentration upon sodium, water, diuretics and the kidneys to concentration upon nutrition and hepatic dysfunction.

Case Reports

Case 1

V. R., a twenty-five-year-old gravida 3, para 0, of thirty-four weeks gestation, was admitted to Jackson Memorial Hospital, April 15, 1960, from a county clinic because of massive edema associated with a 12 lb weight gain in eleven days. The blood pressure was 184/104 with four-plus proteinuria. She had had ankle edema for three weeks and headaches throughout pregnancy. On three previous prenatal clinic visits, the blood pressure had been borderline, 118/90 on March 11, 118/84 on March 25, and 122/88 on April 1, but there was no proteinuria. On March 25, she had been advised to go on a 1,000 cal diet. For two weeks prior to admission, she had eaten practically nothing because of a reactive depression caused by her mother's death. On April 1, she was started on 250 mg chlorothiazide, orally, per day.

This patient was 4 fcet, 10 inches toll and weighed 182 lbs. She had massive generalized edema. The blood pressure was 170/110, temperature normal, pulse, 80; respirations, 20. The heart and lungs were normal. The estimated fetal weight was 2,200 gm, and fetal heart tones were normal.

Laboratory data on admission. Hemoglobin level was 13.4; hematocrit, 43; urinalysis, 960 mg% protein, 5 to 15 white blood cells per high-power field (centrifuged specimen) and many hyaline casts; blood urea nitrogen level, 11.9 mg%; serum uric acid, 8.1 mg%; alkaline phosphatase, 6.1 BU; serum sodium 139; potassium 4.5; and carbon dioxide combining power, 15.5 mEq per liter. On the fourth hospital day total serum protein was 4.42 gm%; with albumin, 1.38 gm%; and globulins, 3.04 gm%, by serum protein electrophoresis.

The patient was treated initially with intravenous chlorothiazide, pentobarbital, diphenylhydantoin and intramuscular magnesium sulfate. The diuretics she received each twenty-four hours from April 15 through April 20, were chlorothiazide 250 mg, 500 mg, 500 mg, 250 mg, 750 mg, and 500 mg plus meralluride, respectively. Her blood pressure remained 140 to 150/90 to 100. Because diuretics were ineffective in mobilizing the edema fluid, they were discontinued on the fifth hospital day and 1,000 cc 5 per cent mannitol was administered. This osmotic diuretic brought about a moderate increase in urinary output but the patient remained massively edematous. Serum sodium dropped from 138 mEq per liter on admission to 128 the next day, to 132 on the third day and to 131 on the fifth day.

Several attempts were made to induce labor with oxytocin drip but all were unsuccessful. On the tenth hospital day, during an oxytocin induction, the fetal heart tones dropped to 90, and a Caesarean section was done immediately with delivery of a healthy 2,350 gm premature infant who survived. Marked diuresis began within two hours following delivery.

The postoperative course was complicated by fluctuating diastolic hypertension for a week postpartum and a urinary tract infection which responded to chloramphenicol. The patient was discharged asymptomatic on the ninth postoperative day with normal blood pressure. On a following-up visit to the clinic on the twenty-first day, her blood pressure was 130/76.

Case 2

C. H., a nineteen-year-old primigravida, was transferred to Jackson Memorial Hospital on July 21, 1960, at thirty-eight weeks gestation, with a history of generalized edema for four weeks and severe headaches and epigastric pain for several days. She had been admitted to a smaller county hospital two days previously because of a convulsion on July 19. On two prenatal visits, in February and April, 1960, the blood pressure had been normal and the urine negative for protein. She failed to return for regular prenatal care. The total weight gain was 59 lbs.

On July 19, the blood pressure was 200/150, the weight 288 lbs, and there was marked generalized edema. She had another convulsion after admission to the county hospital that day. The urine showed four-plus protein, and the blood urea nitrogen level was 15.0 mg%. She was treated with intramuscular hydralazine, oral chlorothiazide, and phenobarbital and a 400 mg low-sodium diet. On July 20, the urinary output was only 600 ml, with an intake of 4,613 ml (Table III). The patient was transferred to our hospital on July 21 with a blood pressure of 178/124. She was grossly obese and edematous; temperature, normal; pulse, 110; respirations, 28. The heart and lungs were clear. The estimated fetal weight was 2,400 gm, and fetal heart tones were normal.

Laboratory data on admission. Hemoglobin level was 12.8; hematocrit, 38.5; urinalysis, 10 to 12 white blood cells per high-power field (centrifuged) and 350 mg% protein; blood urea nitrogen level, 28.8 mg%; serum uric acid, 14.4 mg%; creatinine, 2.0 mg%; SGOT, 36 units, total serum proteins, 4.46 gm% with 1.98 gm% albumin and 2.48 gm% globulins by electrophoresis.

The patient was treated with intravenous chlorothiazide, morphine, hydralazine-cryptenamine drip, and intramuscular magnesium sulfate. The blood pressure came down to 150 to 160/90 to 100 and the urinary output on the first day was considered adequate. Table I presents the data of the fluid flow sheet and pertinent follow-up laboratory studies.

TABLE III
DIURETIC THERAPY AND LABORATORY DATA (CASE 2)*

Diuretic (24-hour dose)	Urinary output (ml)	Intake (ml)	Date	BUN (mg %)	Na-K-Cl (mEq/L)	Others
Chlorothiazide, 1.0 gm, orally	1,350	2,600	7/19/60	15		
Chlorothiazide, 1.0 gm, orally	600	4,613	7/20			
Chlorothiazide, 0.5 gm, orally Chlorothiazide, 0.5 gm, intravenously	2,005	3,440	7/21			Hct. 41
Chlorothiazide, 1.0 gm, intravenously	1,655	2,175	7/22	28.8	140-4.0-101	Creatinine 2.0 mg %
Chlorothiazide, 1.0 gm, intravenously Hydrochlorothiazide, 50 mg, orally	855	4,325	7/23	46.3	134-4.35-98	
Chlorothiazide, 0.5 gm, intravenously Meralluride 2.0 cc, intravenously	2,675	2,325	7/24	53.5	125-4.0-95	Hct. 41
Chlorothiazide, 0.25 gm, intravenously	285	1,700	7/25		126-4.96-95.8	Hct. 40

*Patient died at 7:28 P.M. with massive generalized edema persisting.

Oxytocin induction was attempted unsuccessfully on July 22, the second hospital day, and again on July 23 after artificial rupture of the membranes at 10:50 A.M. Fetal heart tones became irregular at 2:25 P.M. and no longer audible after 5:45 P.M., July 23.

On July 24, the blood pressure ranged from 230/110 to 190/80 and the patient was digitalized because of tachycardia. Oxytocin drip was again unsuccessful and the patient developed a low-grade temperature elevation of 101.6° F. (rectal) at 10:00 P.M. She was started on intramuscular tetracycline. She was given morphine and magnesium sulfate throughout the hospital course.

On July 25, the fifth hospital day, oxytocin drip was given from 8:25 A.M. until noon, at which time the blood pressure suddenly dropped from 190/110 to 90/60 and she became comatose. A phenylephrine drip was begun and at 3:00 P.M., a levarterenol bitartrate drip was set up. The blood pressure then was 140/90 with marked reduction in urinary output. A diagnosis of ruptured uterus was made and, at 6:30 P.M., a Caesarean section without anesthesia was done on a moribund patient. A stillborn infant was delivered. The uterus was intact but would not contract and appeared grossly infected, so a subtotal hysterectomy was performed. The patient died in profound shock at 7:28 P.M., immediately postoperatively.

Autopsy revealed a grossly obese woman with massive edema. There were 200 ml of serous fluid in each pleural space. The lungs showed pulmonary edema. The liver was enlarged (3,050 gm) and pale with a yellow-tan discoloration; there were small petechial hemorrhages scattered over the subdiaphragmatic surfaces. The kidneys were enlarged (250 gm and 270 gm) and appeared edematous. The adrenals were normal. The brain showed a small area of subarachnoid hemorrhage over the parietal region of the left cerebral hemisphere.

Histologic study of the kidneys revealed the glomeruli to be somewhat enlarged with a thickening of the capillary tufts characteristic of "membranous glomerulonephritis" often associated with eclampsia. The liver showed patchy areas of subcapsular hemorrhage with disruption of normal architecture and necrosis of scattered individual cells in the areas of hemorrhage which were not confined to the periportal regions. Most of the liver appeared normal except for generalized edema. The adrenals were normal. Sections of the umbilical cord of the fetus showed no perivascular cellular infiltrations. A blood culture drawn from the heart at autopsy produced a micrococcus, coagulase negative. There was no gross or microscopic evidence of significant infection.

Case 3

G. G., thirty-six-year-old gravida 3, para O, of thirty weeks gestation, was admitted to our emergency room on September 5, 1960, because of convulsions and possible head injury on that day. She had made four prenatal visits to a county clinic where the blood pressure had been normal and no proteinuria found on the first three visits. On the last visit, August 8, four weeks prior to admission, the blood pressure was 100/76; voided urine showed a trace of protein, and the hemoglobin level was 10.2 gm.

On admission to the emergency room, the right eye and face were contused; she was disoriented and lethargic, the tongue swollen and edematous. The blood pressure was 196/136; temperature, 99° F. (rectal); pulse, 140; and respirations, 20. There was pitting edema of both lower extremities to the knees. Deep tendon reflexes were hyperactive with ankle clonus. While skull films were being made, the patient had a generalized grand mal seizure which was controlled with intravenous sodium amobarbital. Skull films and neurological examination revealed no evidence of central nervous system injury (a radiologist observed in his report that skull films were incomplete). The lungs were clear, and the heart normal except for tachycardia. The fetal heart tones were normal and the estimated fetal weight was 1,200 gm.

Laboratory data on admission. Hemoglobin level was 13.2 gm; hematocrit, 43; urinalysis, 500 mg% protein, 10 to 15 white blood cells per high-power field (centrifuged), 3 to 12 red blood cells, a few hyaline and granular casts; serum sodium, 133, potassium, 3.5 (eight hours after admission), carbon dioxide combining power, 11.2, chlorides, 99 mEq per liter; nonprotein nitrogen, 19 mg%; blood urea nitrogen level, 7.6 mg%; total serum proteins, 5.0 gm% with 1.94 gm% albumin and 3.04 gm% globulins by electrophoresis.

A chest x-ray was normal, and an electrocardiogram was borderline with slight S-T depression "probably secondary to rate."

On the labor unit, the patient was treated with intravenous chlorothiazide, sodium amobarbital, diphenylhydantoin, intramuscular magnesium sulfate and nasal oxygen. Table IV indicates the diuretic therapy and changes in serum electrolytes. The blood pressure came down to 125 to 130/100 to 110 with a very narrow

TABLE IV

DIURETIC THERAPY AND SERUM ELECTROLYTES (CASE 3)

Date	Time	Diuretic	Na (mEq/L)	K (mEq/L)	Cl (mEq/L)	CO₂ combining power (mEq/L)
9/5/60	10:50 P.M.	Chlorothiazide, 500 mg, intravenously	133	3.5	99.2	11.2
9/6	5:00 A.M.	Chlorothiazide, 500 mg, intravenously	134	3.0	99.2	19.7
9/7			137	4.0		
9/8			129	5.0	97.5	20.6
9/9						
9/10	Delivery					
9/11			138	5.0	106	18.4

pulse pressure and a persistent tachycardia of 130 to 140. The urinary output for the first sixteen hours was 1,510 with an intake of 1,495; a venous cutdown was done.

At 2:00 P.M., September 6, sixteen hours after admission, the patient went into shock with a weak thready pulse and systolic pressure barely palpable at 80 mm Hg; she was cold and clammy and in deep coma with no urinary output for over forty-five minutes (Fig. 16). At 3:00 P.M., she was given 15 gm of salt-poor human serum albumin by push intravenously over a twenty-minute period and ten gm more were dripped in thereafter. Within eight minutes after the beginning of this injection, the blood pressure had risen to 118/96, and urine was seen dripping freely from the catheter. Within forty-five minutes, the output was 175 ml urine; in the next hour it was 330 ml; and the next hour 330 ml. In the sixteen-hour period following the onset of shock, she received 50 gm of salt-poor serum albumin, had an intake of 2,170 ml of intra-

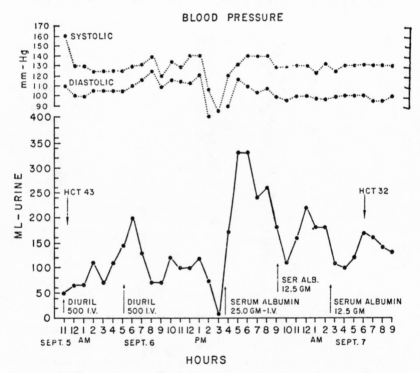

FIGURE 16. Case 3. Urinary output by hours, response to intravenous chlorothiazide and human serum albumin in eclampsia.

venous 5 per cent glucose and excreted 2,858 ml of urine; this urine contained only a "trace" of protein. The edema visibly decreased during this time. At the end of the sixteen-hour period, the hemoglobin had dropped from 13.4 to 8.4 gm and hematocrit from 43 to 32. The pulse slowed to 108 to 112, and blood pressure was stabilized at 130/100 for thirty-eight hours and the output was good. A twenty-four-hour urine specimen, collected from 7:00 A.M., September 6, to 7:00 A.M., September 7, contained 191 mEq sodium, 20 mEq potassium and 174 mEq chloride.

On September 8, the third hospital day, the blood pressure had risen to 150/110 at 8:00 A.M. and she was started on a hydralazine cryptenamine drip. The pulse increased to 120 and urinary output dropped to 50 ml from 9:00 to 10:00 A.M. She was given, by slow drip, 12.5 gm serum albumin at 10:00 A.M., and output increased to 120, 175 and 150 ml in the next three hours. About 1:30 P.M., the patient had an episode of acute bronchospasm and pulmonary edema but responded quickly to treatment with oxygen, rotating tourniquets, intravenous morphine, and aminophylline. She was given digitalis intramuscularly.

On September 9, the fifth hospital day, at 2:00 P.M., she had another episode of bronchospasm without pulmonary edema; this was preceded by a blood pressure elevation to 160/115 for which she received the intravenous hydralazine cryptenamine drip with a subsequent drop to 90/70 and oliguria which lasted for fourteen hours. A blood culture done at this time was later reported to be growing *E. coli;* the diagnosis of septicemia was deemed unlikely. At 9:30 P.M. she was started on intravenous chloramphenicol because of pyuria and evidence that cut-down sites were becoming infected. From 7:00 P.M. until 4:00 A.M. the next day the total urinary output was 70 ml, at this time she went spontaneously into labor. The fetal heart tones could no longer be heard. At 6:35 A.M., on September 10, she was delivered of a 1,600 gm stillborn infant; the urinary output immediately rose to 100 to 200 ml hour. In the twenty-four hours following delivery, the urinary output was 4,410 ml with intake of 2,450 ml.

Postpartum, the patient had a difficult course complicated by a *Staphylococcus aureus* enterocolitis for which she received neomycin orally. The hemoglobin level dropped to 7.8 gm and, she was given 500 ml of whole blood. The cutdown sites healed slowly, and she developed phlebitis of the entire greater saphenous vein in the left leg. The blood pressure remained 150 to 160/90 to 100 for three days and then came down to 140/90. She improved slowly and was discharged on the seventeenth postpartum day asymptomatic. On a clinic visit two weeks later she was doing well and the blood pressure was 110/80.

The above cases illustrate the ineffectiveness of all symptomatic therapies in the woman with severe, life-threatening MTLP. They show the hazards of diuretic therapy and point up the need for rapid delivery of such seriously ill patients. Had we used intravenous albumin in Case 2 and not diuretics, I think she would have survived; if we had delivered her on the second hospital day, both mother and fetus would probably have survived.

A rather extensive literature has accumulated on the use of oral diuretics in prenatal patients and extravagant claims are made that these drugs prevent the development of toxemia. I am certain that these drugs play no such role in the prevention of MTLP. I have seen many women faithfully taking oral saluretic diuretics develop severe MTLP refractory to all therapies except termination of pregnancy. In 1962 Charles Flowers *et. al.,* from Chapel Hill, North Carolina, reported a "double-blind" study on 519 patients on "Chlorothiazide as a Prophylaxis Against Toxemia of Pregnancy," in which they concluded:

1. This study indicates that a group of intelligent patients following prenatal instructions had an insignificant incidence of toxemia and an extremely low perinatal mortality rate.
2. There was no significant difference in the incidence of toxemia between patients who took a diuretic during pregnancy and those who were given a placebo.

It is a commonly known fact in our nation that the severest cases of MTLP are seen in women who have no prenatal care. The fact that a woman presents herself for prenatal care to a physician or public clinic indicates that her level of awareness of the special needs and problems of pregnancy is higher than that of the woman who remains at home until signs or symptoms of the disease cause her to seek medical care.

I have reached the conclusion that saluretic diuretics are actually contra-indicated in pregnancy, except in those cases complicated by cardiovascular or renal diseases.

CHAPTER 7

PRINCIPLES OF MANAGEMENT

THE MANAGEMENT of a pregnant woman who has developed metabolic toxemia of late pregnancy can now be based upon a rational foundation provided by our better understanding of its etiology and abnormal physiology and biochemistry. We need no longer aim blindly at the signs and symptoms of the disease process.

Each case must be individualized and studied carefully. When mild MTLP develops it is possible to correct it by simply encouraging the patient to increase her intake of high biological quality protein. This should be done in the hospital where the patient may be observed carefully. Mild sedation with small doses of phenobarbital may be helpful. There is no rational basis for the use of saluretic diuretics nor anti-hypertensive drugs.

Severe MTLP manifested by toxic symptoms of headaches, nausea, vomiting, scotomata, abdominal pain, anorexia and serious signs such as convulsions, coma, hypovolemia with hemoconcentration, pulmonary edema, etc. is a life-threatening disease. For many years it has been known that delivery is the best therapy for such patients, and it will continue to be the best therapy. When you consider that such women have a severe underlying hepatic dysfunction, are severely malnourished, and that their livers may be the site of fatty infiltration or hemorrhagic necrosis, you can then understand the hazards of procrastination and symptomatic therapies. Diuretics are contraindicated in such women. Infusions of human serum albumin have been useful in combating the hypovolemia and hemoconcentration, and should be used as an emergency measure to prepare the patient for delivery. In our experience, premature labor is common in severe MTLP, and the cervix is often "ripe" long before term.

Therefore most patients with severe MTLP can be induced with an intravenous drip of dilute oxytocin solution after stripping the membranes. In the rare case, Caesarean section may be required when oxytocin induction fails in two or three attempts over a twenty-four to thirty-six-hour period. Whenever it is possible to rupture the membranes without harming the fetus, this should be done, and the patient must be delivered within twenty-four hours after such amniotomy to avoid hazards of intrauterine infection.

It is essential that the severely toxemic patient not be allowed to remain in the labor unit for several days undelivered with the only source of nutrition intravenous glucose.

Sedation of the central nervous system may be accomplished during a convulsion with small doses of intravenous amytal. Magnesium sulfate has been widely used to depress hyperactive reflexes, but its real value is still open to question. It is important not to oversedate these women with drugs such as morphine and the barbiturates which depend upon liver detoxication for their inactivation.

Mengert and Tweedie have recently published good results from following this classical clinical teaching regarding early delivery in severe toxemia. My work offers a scientific rationale for their empirical results.

CHAPTER 8

PREVENTION THROUGH PRENATAL NUTRITIONAL EDUCATION

Hamlin of Australia became convinced of the role of malnutrition in causing toxemia of pregnancy; he gave lectures to women in his prenatal clinics at the Women's Hospital, Sydney, with a remarkable lowering in the incidence of severe MTLP. His theory was based on the idea that Australian women were eating *too much carbohydrate,* and in his efforts to reduce their carbohydrate intake, he encouraged them to take in more high biological quality proteins. In his lectures he used such statements as: "Visit the butcher and not the baker!" and "Put down the bread knife and pick up the butcher knife." Hamlin gave the lectures himself because he realized the importance of *authority* as a psychological force in altering adult human behavior. For this reason I think it is important at this time for a physician to give the prenatal nutrition lectures whenever possible.

With strong clinical, physiological and biochemical evidence that metabolic toxemia of late pregnancy is directly caused by malnutrition during pregnancy, I began in July, 1963, a clinical research project in our county prenatal clinic at Richmond, California. My challenge was not only to tell the pregnant women what they should be eating, but to tell them in such an effective way that they would actually alter their dietary habits and follow out the instructions in daily life. To accomplish this I began giving a group lecture each week to those prenatal patients visiting the clinic for the first visit. Then with each individual patient on her subsequent visits (and I see about one half of all prenatal patients for their regular follow-up visits) I would reinforce the initial educational lecture with questions concerning how well she was following the prescribed diet and also encouraging her at each visit to eat more high biological quality protein foods within the range of her economic limitations. To attempt to give some scientific answer to the question: How does prenatal care as practiced in the United States today lower the incidence of toxemia and other complications? I have not used diuretics nor salt restriction in these patients except on two occasions. I have not stressed to the patient the importance of "total weight gain" but rather stressed consistently the importance of good nutrition. The following is the basic text of the lecture to a group of new prenatal patients on their first clinic visit each Monday morning for the past twenty-six months.

Good morning, I'm Doctor Brewer in obstetrics. I want to spend a few minutes talking with you about your diet in pregnancy. Why? Because eating a good, well-balanced diet during pregnancy is the most important thing you can do to help us help you to have a healthy pregnancy and a healthy, strong baby.

Why do I want to talk to you about diet in pregnancy? Well, for many years I worked with pregnant women in the South, in the city-county hospitals like Charity Hospital, New Orleans, Louisiana, and Jackson Memorial Hospital, Miami, Florida. There I saw a large number of women suffering severe complications of pregnancy such as high blood pressure, swelling, abnormal bleeding, premature deliveries. I became convinced from talking to these women and from doing some chemical studies on their blood that most of their troubles came from not eating the right kind of diet when they got pregnant.

What was wrong with their diets? The main thing that was wrong was that they didn't have enough milk, eggs and meat, the so-called "protein" foods that you especially need when you're pregnant. Many of the women I talked with at Charity Hospital in New Orleans had only one kind of meat in their diets and it was this:

(I take from a paper bag a piece of salt pork and hold it up.) This is salt pork, or "fat back" and if you look at it real carefully, you can see a tiny streak of lean there, but mainly it is nothing but a chunk of fat. These poor women ate this cooked with greens, beans, black-eyed peas. I'm not saying it doesn't taste good or even that it hurts you to eat it once in a while—but it is bad if it's the only kind of meat you have in your diet. So many of these women I talked with had *no lean meat, no eggs, no milk at all* in their diets. A lot of them ate laundry starch and river clay, too.

Well, what should you be eating when you're pregnant?

(I take from the same paper bag a small carton of dry nonfat skim milk and hold it up.)

Milk is one of the most important foods you can take when you're pregnant. Why? Well, milk is a food that Nature provides for young growing things, baby animals, and it has nearly all the food substances in the right amounts that a baby needs to grow up strong. The baby inside you growing now was formed from the union of a sperm cell with a tiny egg from your ovary, and in three months or so it grows into a tiny human baby, and for the last six months of your pregnancy it simply has to grow up inside your womb until it weighs seven or eight pounds and is ready to be born.

The baby growing inside your womb gets its food from your blood stream by means of the placenta, or "afterbirth," where little loops of the baby's blood vessels are bathed in your blood, and the food substances from your blood pass over into the baby's blood vessels and then into its body. It seems a matter of common sense that if you drink a quart of milk every day, you will be feeding the baby inside you a good food for it to grow up healthy and strong. You don't have to drink this dry skim milk, you can drink any kind of milk but it must be a quart every day. I show you this dry skim milk because it is the cheapest kind of good protein food you can buy; if you buy a big box of it, you can get a quart of milk for about eight cents. How many of you already drink a quart of milk every day?

What else besides a quart of milk do you need to eat every day when you're pregnant?

(I take from the same paper bag two chicken eggs.)
You ought to eat *two eggs* every day. An egg has in it all the food substances that a tiny chick embryo needs to grow up into a complete baby chicken; it is probably even a better food than milk. It has some of the best proteins and iron. How many of you eat two eggs every day? If you don't particularly like milk or eggs, you should eat them like they were medicine when you're pregnant, and also when you nurse your baby.

Besides a quart of milk and two eggs every day, you ought to eat lean meat twice a day, a green leafy vegetable and a yellow or red vegetable every day and some kind of citrus fruit or juice like an orange or grapefruit or lemon every day. In general you ought to eat a well-balanced diet and not eat too much fatty foods nor too many sweets nor drink too much pop. Cheese is a good source of protein, especially cottage cheese.

Now there are a few special problems that often come up to keep you from eating a good diet during pregnancy.

1. Many women have morning sickness in early pregnancy but it passes away after a few weeks. If it doesn't, you tell us about it in the clinic and we'll give you some medicine to help. Then about six or seven months along, many pregnant women begin to have heartburn, indigestion, nausea, vomiting. If any of these symptoms come up, be sure to tell us because we want you to have this good diet right up to the day you go into labor.

2. During the last month of pregnancy, as the baby is getting to be fairly big, you may find that your stomach doesn't hold as much as before. We had a woman in here not long ago who gave birth to twins, and each weighed seven and one half pounds. You can imagine how crowded her stomach was. If you need to, you can eat six or eight small meals during the day and even a snack when you wake up in the middle of the night.

3. Some of you may be a little on the heavy side and may be put on a diet. If this happens, don't forget that you still need the quart of milk, two eggs, lean meat, vegetables and fruit every day no matter what other people tell you. Your baby growing inside you can't afford to diet, and you have to furnish it the right foods every day just like you have to feed it properly after it's born. Also if your feet start to swell (and this happens in about 50 per cent of normal women) at some time during your pregnancy, you may be put on a low salt diet. Again remember that even if you cut back on salt and salty foods, you still need these good foods we've been talking about for the baby.

When I came out here to the San Francisco Bay Area, I found that women are generally better off than in the South. Complications of pregnancy aren't so common, but when they do occur, it is usually possible to find that the woman for some reason hasn't been eating a good diet. I want to tell you about one young woman whom I saw in our county hospital in San Francisco while I was working at the University of California.

She was twenty years old and she came here from a foreign country to go to college. She lived with a family and helped look after their children during the day and went to college at night. She wasn't married, and when she got pregnant, she was very ashamed. She decided to hide her pregnancy as long as possible by starving herself. Instead of drinking a quart of milk every day as she should have, she only had one cup of milk three times a week. And she ate no meat and not an egg; she ate vegetables, potatoes and rice. Toward the last part of her pregnancy she began to swell, but she still didn't seek any prenatal care.

When she went into labor, the family called an ambulance. On the way into the hospital in the ambulance she had a fit, a convulsion, which is one of the signs of toxemia of pregnancy she had developed. Her baby delivered shortly after she reached the hospital, and it died. We treated her for the toxemia and she got well in a few days. It was while she was recovering from the toxemia that she told me the story I just told you. When I told her how important good diet and prenatal care are for the pregnant woman, she promised never to do such a foolish thing again.

I'm not trying to frighten you; it is just that I have seen so many young women like this trying to hide their pregnancies, not eating right, not coming to prenatal clinics when they get pregnant, that I want you to profit from their unfortunate experiences. Pregnancy, in general, today is a very healthy state for women who eat right and get prenatal care. If you eat right and keep your clinic appointments, you'll have the best chances of having a strong, healthy baby and of staying in good health yourself. Are there any questions about your diet in pregnancy?

If you have any questions that come up during your pregnancy or any special problems about your diet, be sure to tell us during your clinic visits. You already have been given some vitamin capsules and some iron tablets to take, but let me emphasize that the best vitamins you get are in a well-balanced diet and the best iron is in meat and eggs. Remember, a quart of milk every day, two eggs every day, and lean meat twice a day are so important for you to have a healthy, strong, full-term baby and to stay healthy yourself.

This is so important that if it happens that there is an extra piece of meat on the table at supper after you've all been served ... and later your husband reaches for it, tell him: "Wait a minute, I'm pregnant and I'm supposed to have that. The doctor said so; he told me to tell you that you can have another potato but that I need the meat specially."

Thank you.

On follow-up visits I ask each of my patients if she has been following the diet as discussed in the lecture, and I encourage her to eat better when it's indicated. The results of this program have been excellent. Approximately one thousand patients have heard the lecture, and not one case of severe metabolic toxemia of late pregnancy has developed in our clinic patients. In the first 235 patients who have delivered and whose hospital records I have studied, there has been no MTLP. Seven patients developed a mild hypertension while in labor which subsided within six to forty-eight hours postpartum. Four patients developed proteinuria associated with a urinary tract infection, and there was no other proteinuria. There have been four infants under 2500 gm (one of these had a twin which was over 2500 gm) and only one premature weighed under 1800 gm. There was one 234 gm macerated stillborn. This premature rate is less than 2 per cent.

These women in my clinic are on the bottom of the socioeconomic scale, and over 50 per cent of them are Negroes. In the group of 235 patients delivered, seventy-three were primiparous, many only fourteen, fifteen and sixteen years of age, yet not one developed MTLP. Among a similar group of primiparous patients delivered at Jackson, Mississippi, in the University of Mississippi Hospital, 35 per cent developed toxemia (Michael Newton, 1964). It is scientific to conclude that when every pregnant woman in Mississippi has adequate nutrition, metabolic toxemia of late pregnancy will disappear as it has among my prenatal patients at the Richmond Health Center in Richmond, California.

CHAPTER 9

"HIGH RISK" PATIENTS

For many physicians in private practice of obstetrics here in the United States there are few problems concerning nutrition in pregnancy. Private obstetricians from ten states have told me that they encounter a very low incidence of toxemia, toxic abruptio placentae and other complications which concern us here. However, many private obstetricians take responsibilities at city-county and teaching hospitals where they do come in contact with these problems and where they exert influence on medical students, interns and residents.

The following discussion is presented to remind the reader that certain common clinical conditions frequently develop which tend to interfere with good prenatal nutrition. Whenever the physician encounters such patients, he must be particularly alert and take every action possible to correct the clinical problem and to insure good nutrition. This discussion is not intended to be an exhaustive and authoritative dissertation on the various problems presented rather briefly; it is intended to further strengthen the point of view that pregnancy is a condition in which every effort must be made to maintain adequate nutrition in the face of clinical complications and socioeconomic obstacles. The recognition of these problems is the first prerequisite for their effective solution.

THE IMPORTANCE OF A GOOD CLINICAL HISTORY IN OBSTETRICAL PRACTICE AND RESEARCH

Obstetrics is one of the broadest specialities, for in it one is concerned with practically every disorder except those peculiarly male. It is medicine and it is surgery, and it is psychiatry. The individual obstetrician may lean closer to a surgical outlook than to a medical outlook. No matter what our individual orientation, in order to really practice good obstetrics, we must continue to apply those techniques taught us with so much devotion and enthusiasm by our professors and instructors of internal medicine in the art and science of history-taking. For it is only by a complete history that we can really get a clear understanding of our patients, and it is only by an accurate and thorough history that we can make sense out of the vast amount of laboratory data we are able to gather in the modern hospital or outpatient clinic. And on the scientific foundation furnished by a good history we can plan our management of the individual patient so much more rationally.

A clear picture of the historical background of a patient will also aid the physician who wishes to do clinical research, for he will be able to ask the right questions of Nature, and he will avoid certain errors made by the authorities who preceded him in the human struggle for scientific knowledge. It was from the clinical histories of dozens of poor women living in our southern states that I became convinced of the significance of the role of malnutrition in the pathogenesis of metabolic toxemia of late pregnancy. It was from these histories that I was able to understand the physiological significance of hypoalbuminemia, hypovolemia and hemoconcentration in these severely ill women and the hazards of diuretic therapy. And it was from these histories that I was able to plan a successful program of prevention through prenatal nutritional education among clinic patients to test the theory.

Modern biochemistry has much to offer clinical medicine, but at present it is not clinically oriented. It has its own history, traditions and scientific outlook, but it is forging the tools for clinical investigators who must come firmly to grips with many unsolved clinical problems. The current popular interest in superscientific computers, in complex laboratory instruments, in radioisotopes must not turn us away from our basic clinical tool: the history of the patient. Nor should these products of the physical sciences blind us to the socioeconomic and historical realities of our culture, to the unsatisfactory human conditions from which we now know so many of the complications of pregnancy arise. It is *out there,* away from our clean hospitals and modern scientific laboratories loaded with precision machines of scientific research, that human diseases have their origin. We must go *out there* to really understand our patients, and the chief tool we have at present to recapture the individual and unique past of our patients is the clinical history.

THE TEEN-AGE MOTHER-TO-BE

I am convinced that there is nothing about teen-age pregnancy, *per se,* that causes difficulty. I have cared for hundreds of such young mothers-to-be who sailed through pregnancy, labor and delivery without batting an eye. The problem which faces us is that so many of these young women in the lowest socioeconomic class don't come in for adequate prenatal care. They also have eating habits which are far from optimal when they're not pregnant. I have discussed this with nutritionists and dieticians from a number of different institutions, and there seems to be a consensus of opinion that these young women as a group do not have good nutrition. Many of them are immature with no significant knowledge of biology nor of physiology, and they live in a world very different from the worlds of the health authorities who are trying to help them. They are also frequently unmarried, live in large families where there may be already too many mouths to feed, and they may come under considerable psychological stress during pregnancy. Whenever a teen-age girl comes to a physician or public prenatal clinic, special efforts should be made to contact some responsible adult in her family and to educate both the patient and the adult as to the importance of good nutrition in pregnancy. I have seen four twelve-year-olds deliver babies, and they are hardly old enough to be responsible for themselves; the same may be said for many of the thirteen-fourteen- and fifteen-year old mothers-to-be.

THE "UNWED MOTHER"

Social scientists, social workers, educators, legal authorities, public health authorities are increasingly concerned with the problem of the "unwed mother." The discussion presented above about teen-age pregnancy applies here, but of course many older women have this problem. I have seen so much sorrow and difficulty and pregnancy complications arise out of these situations that I make a plea here for more kindness and understanding in our society and in our approach to these patients. One striking phenomenon occurs frequently in our society: a woman who is "illegitimately" pregnant will attempt to hide her pregnancy as long as possible by starving herself, and this can have disastrous results. Sometimes the attitude of the patient's family can cause her great difficulty as in the folowing case. An older woman came into the labor unit at Jackson Memorial Hospital, the city-county hospital in Miami, Florida, for delivery. She told the labor nurses about her seventeen-year-old neighbor who was about six months pregnant and unmarried. The older woman had tried to convince the young woman to come into our prenatal clinic but without success. The young woman's family was very unkind to her and often gave her the scraps from their table. They would on occasions lock her out of the house at night. One evening the older woman had met the young woman going to the store with a dime in her hand to buy her supper.

The labor nurses noted the girl's name; about four weeks later she was admitted to our labor unit with severe metabolic toxemia of late pregnancy. Here we had an unusual observation into the life of a toxemic patient, a view which might not have been recorded by the usual obstetrical history.

As a general rule those women who go to a home for unwed mothers such as those operated by the Salvation Army and the Florence Crittenden Homes fare much better. If they stay in these institutions any significant length of time prior to delivery, they have access to very good prenatal nutrition. Dodek of George Washington University, Washington, D.C., reported in 1960 that among 300 patients seventeen years old and younger in Florence Crittenden Homes in that city, only two patients developed toxemia of late pregnancy. Officials of two Salvation Army maternity homes have told me that their incidence of toxemia is very low. There seems to be no doubt that the unwed mother needs kindness and good food.

WOMEN IN POVERTY: TOO MANY MOUTHS TO FEED

All over the world women in the lower socioeconomic classes suffer the most and most severe complications of pregnancy. Bryan Hibbard of Liverpool, who has found a constant relationship between folic acid deficiency and the occurrence of abruptio placentae has written these words recently.

> Diet cannot be judged by calories alone and it is likely that *mal*nutrition rather than *under*nutrition is far more common in Great Britain than is realized. Reduction of the hazards associated with

pregnancy anaemia, with abruption and with abortion lies in some measure in the long-term policy of health education and social reform which will result in vitamins being bought not from the pharmacy but from the butcher and the greengrocer.

Do American physicians generally realize how much malnutrition exists here in the United States? Jean Mayer, Professor of Nutrition, Harvard School of Public Health, has recently published a startling report on the food habits and nutritional status of American Negroes. He reports that 60 per cent of Negro families and 25 per cent of Caucasian families in our southern states have "obviously inadequate diets." This article gives an up-to-date background for my research work carried on many years in our southern states, where I learned from the study of hundreds of women living in poverty of the role that malnutrition plays in the pathogenesis of metabolic toxemia of late pregnancy. The death rate from this disease has been consistently five times higher in "non-white" pregnant women than in "white" pregnant women for many years.

I visited in the homes of several of our eclamptic patients and found overcrowding, family disorganization, low education level and alcoholism. One of our eclamptic patients took her infant from the hospital nursery into a three-room shack where the infant made the thirteenth person living there. These are the culture media in which eclampsia flourishes. It is my firm opinion that as obstetricians we have a public responsibility to convey to the American people and to our political authorities the scientific data which so clearly indicate the roles of poverty and malnutrition in producing many of the major complications of pregnancy. It will then become the responsibility of the entire society to insure that all American women get adequate prenatal care and adequate diets when they become pregnant.

EATING FOR THREE: TWIN GESTATION

It is widely accepted that multiple pregnancy is associated with a higher incidence of a host of complications of pregnancy, including metabolic toxemia of late pregnancy, hydramnios, prematurity and anemia. Much emphasis has been placed by certain authorities on "uterine overdistention" produced by the increased number of fetuses. Since the large majority of twin gestations are *not* associated with MTLP, it seems reasonable to suspect that factors other than uterine overdistention are at work in this disease, which is common in single-fetus pregnancies. It is obvious that a twin pregnancy imposes a greater nutritional burden on a woman. If she has a borderline diet, the extra fetus can readily enhance the state of nutritional deficiency. A twin gestation usually is associated with a *larger placenta,* which produces more steroid hormones for the liver to detoxify. Bengtsson and Ejarque have recently reported a woman with twin gestation whose placental production of progesterone in a twenty-four-hour period was calculated from isotope dilution techniques to be 520 mgm. We are accustomed to think of 100 mgm of progesterone as a potent physiological dose.

It has been shown that hospitalization during the last trimester improves the obstetrical performance of women with multiple pregnancies and lowers their premature rate. I think that the improved nutrition made available to such women in the hospital plays a significant role in this. While it may not be practical or necessary to hospitalize such women with multiple pregnancy, it is important to emphasize to each woman the importance of her taking a good diet with emphasis on high biological quality proteins and vitamins, contained in fresh vegetables. Once the unscientific fear of "obesity" and "weight gain" is banished, the physician will feel more comfortable and certain in telling the woman with twins to "eat for three."

FOOD HABITS, FADS AND FOOLISH NOTIONS

Food habits are among the most highly conditioned of human activities. While biochemistry divides foods into simple categories, the world of human culture presents endless complexities and varieties, and there are a thousand and more opinions about what is "good food" and what is not. During my years of medical work in the southern states, I was amazed at the number of pregnant women who said to me: "I don't like milk; it sours on my stomach!" or "Milk makes me sick!" "I don't like eggs . . . ugh!" (Almost as if the thought of "eggs" were itself nauseating.) "I don't like meat." This latter was most difficult for me to accept, but I have heard it from dozens and dozens of pregnant women, particularly from those in whom serious complications developed. Nearly every woman has some fruit or vegetable which she actively "dislikes," and for some it is a very long list. The nutritional status of a patient can never be taken for granted; an awareness of these "likes" and "dislikes" will help make the clinical dietary history more accurate and meaningful.

Ferguson and Keaton in 1950 reported quite a number of women living in Mississippi who ate river clay and laundry starch while pregnant. Many living in New Orleans would return to their native rivers to bring back boxes of clay to eat throughout pregnancy. Some would consume as much as three boxes of "Argo" starch a day, though usually they ate just the lumps. Among women in the San Francisco Bay Area who have come from our southern states, I still frequently encounter women who eat a significant amount of laundry starch. Seldom will a woman volunteer the information that she is eating starch; you have to ask her and advise against it. She usually learned about eating starch from her mother, grandmother, aunts or sisters. Occasionally one encounters a profound nutritional anemia among women eating large amounts of starch.

Not infrequently, one encounters a pregnant woman who has the idea that she is "allergic" to a host of good foods such as milk, eggs, meat, many fruits. This may impose a problem, and every effort should be made to correct the patient's irrational ideas so that they don't interfere with good nutrition. Many young women eat large amounts of candy, cakes, potato chips and drink large quantities of soda pop. When they become pregnant it is necessary to make a real effort to change these poor habits of nutrition. It is for this reason that I inquire of each patient at each prenatal visit about her diet and encourage her to eat the right things. It is only by this constant repetition that long-standing habits can be changed. This is the nature of the human nervous system that Pavlov began to study. An awareness of the role of "conditioning" in human behavior will aid the obstetrician in understanding his patient and in helping her change her unhealthy food habits.

DIABETES MELLITUS

Before the advent of insulin it was rare for a woman with severe diabetes mellitus to deliver a viable infant; today there are still "brittle" juvenile diabetics who have much difficulty with or without pregnancy. For a large number of women, insulin, proper diet and antibiotics have made pregnancy relatively safe for the woman, and the practice of preterm induction of labor has improved the fetal outcome even more.[57] In no other disease state is good nutrition more important than in the pregnant diabetic woman. Garfield Duncan once said at a medical meeting that he believed that he was preventing toxemia of pregnancy by good management of diabetes during pregnancy. He advocated that each pregnant diabetic woman have 2.0 gm of protein per kg body weight as a base.

We know from experience that the poorly controlled or neglected diabetic will develop MTLP, a fatty liver, be more susceptible to infections (particularly to urinary tract infections) develop acidosis and ketosis and that her baby will die several weeks before term. She will be more prone to develop hydramnios. Preterm delivery is the accepted method of management for all diabetics, mild or severe, because intrauterine fetal deaths occur too frequently in spite of therapy.

It is important to stress the role of high biological quality proteins in the diet of the pregnant diabetic. Both internist and dietician can be of considerable help to the obstetrician, because diabetes mellitus well managed has a much lower association with MTLP. The common association of MTLP with the malnourished diabetic is further evidence in my mind that toxemia is a disease of metabolic nature caused by nutritional deficiency. There is no scientific basis for the use of progesterone and estrogens in pregnant diabetics, and it is possible that such therapy could be harmful to both mother and fetus.

GI BLUES: PERNICIOUS VOMITING, DIAPHRAGMATIC HERNIA, ESOPHAGITIS, PEPTIC ULCER SYNDROME, THE CROWDED STOMACH

The gastrointestinal tract undergoes certain changes during pregnancy. Being made up primarily of smooth muscle, it loses some of its tone like other smooth muscle in the body (especially in the ureters) under the influence of the placental hormones. As pregnancy advances it becomes crowded as the expanding uterus encroaches on its living space within the abdomen; this may be particularly marked with multiple pregnancy, a large single fetus or hydramnios. These mechanical factors may interfere with nutrition.

The common nausea of early pregnancy, the so-called "morning sickness," usually lasts only a few weeks. Rarely will it persist for months and offer a real challenge to the physician. When nausea and vomiting are so marked that the patient fails to gain weight and becomes dehydrated, the diagnosis of "pernicious vomiting of pregnancy" is entertained. This clinical situation is usually associated with one of three conditions: hepatitis; hydatid mole; and psychoneurosis or psychosis. The use of intravenous glucose and electrolytes and vitamins is well established. Infusions of human serum albumin may be useful to replenish protein stores and to provide daily protein needs. The patient under psychic stress often benefits by hospitalization in which she is temporarily isolated from the precipitating causes of her emotional stress.

At six to seven months gestation many women begin to have upper GI symptoms related to a diaphragmatic hernia with an associated esophagitis. It is surprising how often it is possible to obtain a past history of such GI distress during pregnancy from older women with diaphragmatic hernias. Antacids, antispasnodics, frequent feedings and elevation of the head of the bed on six-inch blocks will often bring considerable relief to these women. It is important that the problem be aggressively treated so that adequate prenatal nutrition can be maintained. It is also important that the woman not ingest large quantities of antacids like aluminum hydroxide just before or just after meals, because this can interfere with enzymatic digestion of dietary proteins in the stomach and with absorption of amino acids from the small bowel.

Out of many years of general practice there is no question in my mind but that the "peptic ulcer syndrome" is a "psychosomatic" disorder. It is one of the most common disorders that brings a younger person to a physician in the United States, and it is very common among our people at all ages. A skilled physician can nearly always find out the *problem situation* which has precipitated the symptoms, though of course the basic causes lie in early experiences in infancy and childhood. Young women who are pregnant are often under emotional stress of some sort, and they frequently have upper GI distress related to this. Treatment with antacids and antispaomodics is not enough for these patients; they must be "listened to" and supported in their efforts to solve their problems. An understanding obstetrician or general practitioner can usually manage these patients, though at times the consultation of a psychiatrist is required. Again it is urgent that the GI symptoms be relieved or palliated to a degree that good nutrition can be maintained throughout pregnancy.

Mechanical factors, as mentioned above, may crowd the stomach so that the patient is only able to eat small amounts at a time; she fills up quickly. A solution to this problem is frequent small meals throughout the day and a nighttime snack when she awakes at 2:00 or 3:00 A.M. Where there's a will, there's a way. We are determined to let no obstacle stand in the way of achieving good nutrition for our pregnant patients.

MEDICAL PROBLEMS

These conditions are mentioned because they may throw some additional nutritional burden on the pregnant woman. It is very clear from recent reports that good prenatal care and good nutrition will prevent serious complications of pregnancy in women with chronic hypertension and nephritis.[58, 59] Here we must keep in mind that salt restriction must not interfere with good protein intake. In the nephrotic syndrome which rarely occurs in pregnancy, a woman may lose as much as 30 gm of protein daily in her urine; this will present quite a challenge.

Women with active liver diseases seldom get pregnant, but pregnant women may develop hepatitis. Studies reported from Israel and India have shown that well-nourished women have a much better prognosis with viral hepatitis than malnourished women. For a number of years certain obstetrical authorities have ignored the problem of hepatic function in the pathogenesis of toxemia of late pregnancy because women with cirrhosis of the liver who get pregnant usually do well and don't get toxemia. It is important to remember that a necessary prerequisite to pregnancy in these women is a fairly normal liver function which returns after they quit drinking and start eating a balanced diet. They usually get prenatal medical care and are thus protected from the severe malnutrition experienced by our poor women in city and rural slums.

In 1957 C.C. Draa of the University of Illinois presented a report in Chicago on 600 pregnant women with active pulmonary tuberculosis who were treated in Cook County sanitaria from 1945 to 1955. From this experience he learned that tuberculosis does not alter the outcome of pregnancy in any way detrimental to the mother or to the fetus. In general his patients did very well indeed. They were treated exactly like the nonpregnant patients with tuberculosis: proper isolation; rest; good nutrition; proper patient education about the problem; antimicrobial therapy (which consisted of Isoniazid 5 mgm per kilogram body weight per day in three divided doses, streptomycin 1.0 gm intramuscularly twice weekly and PAS 12.0 gm daily in divided doses) and surgery when indicated. A remarkable result was obtained among these 600 women: there was *not a single case* of severe metabolic toxemia of late pregnancy, and only ten patients developed "mild toxemia." When one considers that these women were from the lowest socioeconomic class in county institutions, one can see immediately the dramatic effects of improving their "cultural environment," of feeding them a decent diet.

MENTAL AND EMOTIONAL PROBLEMS: EPILEPSY, PSYCHONEUROSIS, PSYCHOSIS, ALCOHOLISM, NARCOTIC ADDITION, THE WANDERING HUSBAND, THE HUSBAND IN JAIL

Any disorder of the central nervous system, of functional or organic nature, which interferes with rational thought and action and with normal self-protective functions, may interfere with a patient's nutrition during pregnancy. In the course of working years in our public clinics, I have observed so many women under all types of emotional stress. In a busy prenatal clinic it is sometimes difficult for the physician to look at each patient as an individual but nevertheless this is our challenge if we want to be first-class physician-obstetricians and not just technicians.

Simple questions about the patient's family, home, daily experiences, sleep patterns, will quickly reveal those who are grappling with overwhelming personal problems. A history or clinical record of the patient's having tried to abort herself is particularly significant. Epilepsy may be a distressing problem and the patient needs more than the usual support from her obstetrician. Most emotionally stressed pregnant women can be managed by an aware obstetrician, but patients with severe psychoneurotic and psychotic reactions need to be under the care of a psychiatrist in a mental health clinic or hospital.

Alcoholism disrupts pregnancy when the patient is drinking heavily and not eating right. It is also a common problem for the pregnant woman when her husband is drinking heavily. The following case is illustrative:

A twenty-two-year-old immigrant woman came into our county

hospital at thirty weeks gestation with no previous prenatal care. She had had no formal education in her native country. She had had two normal, full-term infants prior to the present pregnancy.

She had hypertension, generalized edema and proteinuria in the absence of infection. She gave a history of eating only macaroni and beans throughout this pregnancy. Her husband had a job, but he was drinking heavily on weekends, and she barely had enough money to feed her other two children.

She was treated with phenobarbital, bed rest for one day and then full ambulation and started on the regular hospital diet with no sodium restriction. Within a week she had lost 7 lbs, her edema had disappeared, her blood pressure had returned to normal, and her proteinuria had cleared.

I was able to talk with the patient and her husband about these problems of pregnancy nutrition, and they both promised that if I would let her go home, she would drink at least a quart of milk daily, eat two eggs and lean meat twice a day, as well as fruits and vegetables. The husband promised to stop spending his wages on alcohol and buy food for his wife, and they promised she would attend the clinic regularly until she delivered. The last eight weeks of the patient's pregnancy were perfectly normal, and she delivered a term infant with no difficulty. The infant was healthy and did well. Her blood pressure, even during labor, did not go over 110/70, and she had no more edema nor proteinuria.

Another striking case was a forty-three-year-old primigravida, unmarried, with a history of chronic essential hypertension, who came into our university hospital early in the third trimester with marked hypertension, generalized edema and proteinuria. The father of the infant was of a different racial origin, and although he wanted to marry her, she had refused; so he left her. For several weeks prior to admission she had been staying alone in her apartment drinking over a pint of whiskey each day and eating very poorly. The obstetrical resident's history did not record this important information.

Our prisons are usually filled with young men; there are about 70,000 men in prisons in California now. Many of these men are fathers-to-be. The mothers-to-be so involved with husbands in jail are sometimes left isolated from society and become depressed. It is also not uncommon for a husband to leave his wife when she becomes pregnant; she then has the total responsibility for herself and for any other dependent children in the family. It is particularly important to help these women with psychological and nutritional counseling. It is quite obvious that a pregnant woman addicted to narcotics presents a challenging problem, and we know the fetus can become addicted *in utero*.

PREMATURE LABOR AND DELIVERY

Let us enter the field of speculation. Month after month, year after year in our monthly perinatal mortality conferences at Jackson Memorial Hospital, Miami, Florida, we discussed the stillbirths and neonatal deaths from the point of view of the obstetrician and pediatrician. This hospital serves both "private" patients and "staff" patients. The premature delivery rate was consistently three times higher among the "staff" patients than among the "private" patients. Even when we could account for a number of the prematures associated with severe toxemia, abruptio placentae, placenta praevia, multiple pregnancies, Rh inductions, etc., we were still left with quite a large number of premature deliveries with no recognizable causes. It is among these women that I suspect that malnutrition is playing a fundamental role in causing premature labor and delivery. The premature rate of less than 2 per cent among my clinic patients at Richmond shows what good prenatal nutrition can do even in the present state of our ignorance of the exact mechanisms. Good prenatal nutrition thus can play a role in the prevention of many of the common permanent complications of the premature infant, including cerebral palsy.

CHAPTER 10

"RED HERRINGS" IN "TOXEMIA" RESEARCH

WHY HAS SUCH A common disease as metabolic toxemia of late pregnancy resisted scientific inquiry so long? Part of the answer has been given in Chapter 2, where it is pointed out how this disorder has been studied as a "syndrome" and not clearly identified as a *disease entity.* Indeed, when I was a student in medical school in 1950, there was serious doubt among some internists that there was any such disease as "toxemia of pregnancy." In this work I hope to establish the scientific reality of this often severe metabolic disease. Another part of the answer may be found in certain armchair theories about its pathogenesis which have gripped the minds of most obstetricians and kept them from seeing the forest for the trees. These "trees" which have obscured the scene and actually contributed to the establishment in clinical obstetrics in the United States of unscientific and irrational practices and attitudes concerning prenatal nutrition are the following:

1. "Statistical associations" with a host of clinical phenomena, related to "hypoxia."
2. Toxemia is a kidney disease, related to salt intake somehow.
3. Toxemia is a disease of "placental insufficiency."
4. Toxemia is a disease of overdistention of the uterus.
5. Toxemia is a congenital disease.
6. Toxemia is a disease of psychosomatic origin.
7. Toxemia is related to atmospheric, telluric conditions.

I will discuss each of these in turn and show how they are not based on any real, solid scientific evidence and furthermore, how they actually block further scientific progress in this field. Unless one can free his mind of these unphysiological and unscientific concepts, it will be impossible to understand the basic point of view developed in this book.

"STATISTICAL ASSOCIATIONS"

"Statistical associations" of metabolic toxemia of late pregnancy with a host of clinical phenomena such as primiparity, multiple pregnancy, hydramnios, obesity, familial incidence, chronic hypertension, diabetes mellitus, emotional stress, placental infarcts, have left obstetricians overwhelmed with a vast amount of clinical data out of which they have sought some common thread of understanding. Claude Bernard gives us excellent advice in his *Introduction to the Study of Experimental Medicine,* 1865.

> Experimental criticism should reject statistics as a foundation
> for experimental therapeutic and pathological science.

It is important to study that statement. Bernard didn't reject statistics as a guide to understanding scientific medical problems, but as a materialist, or "rational determinist," he sought to understand the real relationships of physiologic events as they are linked causally in Nature independent of the mind of the human observer. It is important to realize that statistical manipulations of data in clinical medical research are merely ways of thinking about the phenomena in the mind of the researchers. Conclusions reached from such abstract cerebrations may or may not be related to physiological reality.

Ernest Page developed his idea of a primary "utero-placental ischemia (or hypoxia)" to explain these statistical associations about MTLP which had been set down by the obstetrical authorities who preceded him in this field of research.[61] He borrowed the concept advanced by Goldblatt concerning the "ischemic kidney." From the point of view of the homeostasis of the human body as developed by Claude Bernard and Walter Cannon, Goldblatt's concept fits the logic of the body: If a part of the kidney becomes ischemic because of a reduction of blood flow to that part as a *primary event,* then the elaboration of a vasoconstrictor substance, or its precursor, to raise the systemic blood pressure would function to increase the blood flow to the ischemic renal tissue and correct the situation. This fits the concept of homeostasis that the body is in a constant state of change and struggle to maintain its steady state in an indifferent and often hostile external environment.

Page's idea, on the other hand, postulates that the substance, *X,* the alleged vasoconstrictor, produced somewhere in the uterus as the result of a primary reduction of utero-placental blood flow, actually results in a vasospasm which further reduces utero-placental blood flow and leads to even greater "ischemia." This concept is basically illogical and just does not fit with modern conceptions of physiology. Page set out "to prove" his theory by putting clamps on the abdominal aortas of pregnant bitches, and he was able to record some degree of increase in blood pressures in these animals' systemic circulations. Kumar likewise repeated Page's experiments, but he found that he had to practically tie off the entire blood supply to the uterus and ovaries before he could get much of a blood pressure response. Various other investigators have manipulated the blood supply to the uterus in various ways seeking to confirm this idea of "utero-placental ischemia."

All of these experiments have one vital weakness: We never find in Nature, in toxemic women such clamps on the abdominal aortas nor ligatures on the ovarian and uterine arteries. Furthermore, we can not even visualize *how* primiparity, obesity, multiple pregnancy, etc. could produce such a drastic reduction in utero-placental blood flow as that produced by such clamps and ligatures. Another weakness in this basic hypothesis is that there has been no scientific evidence advanced to demonstrate that a primary reduction in utero-placental blood flow *precedes* the onset of vasoconstriction in toxemic women.

Preoccupations with these ideas have brought about some startling results so that Hunter and Howard actually "found" the hypothetical substance, X, postulated by Page, and they named it "hysterotonin." A critical analysis of their data by an objective biochemist indicates that it is meaningless; Page has tried to reproduce their work but failed. Likewise, their clinical data on women whose "toxemia" was dramatically cured by uterine curettage is open to serious question.

During the year I was associated with Dr. Page at the University of California, I was never able to free his mind of this trap of "statistical associations." For this reason he refused to seriously consider my work on the beneficial effects of intravenous infusions of human serum albumin in women with severe MTLP in whom I observed dramatic diureses with expansion of blood volumes and improvement in renal function. He also disregarded the data I had obtained from the clinical histories of hundreds of women in our southern states living in poverty, and he disregarded my work on the effects of neomycin and sulfathalidine to sterilize the GI tracts of toxemic women. He finally came to the point of admitting that poor nutrition might play some "predisposing role" in the pathogenesis of toxemia, but he was never able to trace just what that role could be in terms of his own theory. If we are going to make further scientific progress in understanding the pathogenesis of metabolic toxemia of late pregnancy, we are going to have to abandon this idea of a primary "utero-placental ischemia," because it has no support in recent clinical, physiological, biochemical or pathological or epidemiological studies.

TOXEMIA IS A KIDNEY DISEASE, RELATED TO SALT INTAKE SOMEHOW

Although most obstetrical authorities deny it, they really think of toxemia of pregnancy as a *kidney* disease, because it presents clinically so much like a kidney disease, like glomerulonephritis. Because there has been observed a glomerular lesion in toxemia, because there is proteinuria, a reduction in glomerular filtration, and sodium and water retention, obstetricians formed themselves a "salt club" and placed great emphasis upon dietary salt restriction and the use of saluretic diuretics. They tended to ignore the glaring differences between severe toxemia and a true kidney disease, particularly the extremely low blood volumes in the severe toxemic patient associated with hypoalbuminemia and hemoconcentration. A primary glomerular dysfunction produces an increase in blood volume and not a decrease. The low serum urea nitrogen levels were also ignored. As we discussed in Chapter 4, the internists and renal physiologists have never been interested in toxemia of pregnancy as a kidney disease because it isn't one. The renal manifestations of this disease are the end result of damage to the glomerular endothelial tufts in the nephron as there is such damage widely about the body. In severe MTLP the reduction in glomerular filtration rate is secondary to a primary reduction in renal blood flow, and when this renal blood flow is increased at delivery and with infusions of human serum albumin, the toxemic kidneys function beautifully. If we are going to make scientific progress in understanding this disease we are going to have to shift our attention away from the kidney. (See Table II.)

So carried away with "salt and water retention" have students of this disease become that they have seen "mirages" in the retinae of "toxemic" women and thought they were seeing "water," as a child sees such mirages while riding along the hot dessert highway and thinks "water." Finnerty has described a "retinal sheen" which he claims is pathognomonic for "toxemia of pregnancy" regardless of the presence or absence of all other signs and symptoms of this disease. He believes that this "sheen" represents a "wet retina" and indicates sodium and water retention. Consultation with several competent opthalmologists including Dr. Edward Norton of the University of Miami School of Medicine, about this question has convinced me that this "retinal sheen" which Finnerty claims is "water" is in reality the light from the opthalmoscope reflected from the optical surface where the vitreous is fused to the retina. This phenomenon, according to Dr. Norton, is common in children and young adults and tends to disappear with age as the vitreous slowly contracts and disrupts the optical surface. True edema of the retina gives it a grayish appearance and no "sheen."

TOXEMIA IS A DISEASE OF "PLACENTAL INSUFFICIENCY"

"Placental insufficiency" is a concept that is still very popular among obstetricians because of the common association of placental infarcts with toxemia, and the endocrine studies in which the low excretion of placental steroid metabolites has been interpreted as evidence of a deficiency in placental production of such steroids. These concepts have already been discussed and criticized. There has been no clear-cut association of placental infarcts with MTLP because many women with severe MTLP have been observed to have no such infarcts, while many women with severely infarcted placentas have been observed to have no MTLP. When placental infarcts do occur associated with MTLP, they may scientifically be regarded as the *end result* of the metabolic, nutritional deficiency disease. To keep our interest and attention focused on the uterus and placenta is to remain forever in the dark about the pathogenesis of this disease.

TOXEMIA IS A DISEASE OF OVER-DISTENTION OF THE UTERUS

Overdistention of the uterus has been considered to be one of the causes of "utero-placental ischemia" as well as the cause of a "utero-renal reflex" which is supposed to result in a constriction of the afferent glomerular arterioles (Sophian, 1955). This latter concept faces an insurmountable hurdle in the observed hypovolemia and hemoconcentration of MTLP. The role of uterine overdistention as playing any part in the pathogenesis of MTLP may be set aside for the following reasons.

1. The large majority of women with "over-distended" uteri do *not* develop MTLP. This includes women with multiple pregnancy, large babies, hydramnios.

2. MTLP has been reported in women with extra-uterine pregnancies which were advanced near term.[70, 71]

3. I have observed a patient with MTLP who developed hydramnios three weeks *after* admission to our hospital for treatment of her toxemia. The hydramnios in this woman was the result of the toxemic process and not its cause.[12]

TOXEMIA IS A CONGENITAL DISEASE

"Congenital factors" have been suspected as playing a role in the pathogenesis of MTLP. Any disease with such clear-cut association with poverty and the lowest socioeconomic class and which is a disease of nutritional deficiency will certainly be "familial" in a sociological or cultural sense. Children develop their dietary habits from the people they grow up with. There remains one remote theoretical possibility to explain a rare case: There may be a few cases of MTLP related to congenital deficiencies in hepatic enzyme systems which detoxify aromatic compounds.

TOXEMIA IS A DISEASE OF PSYCHOSOMATIC ORIGIN

In a certain sense psychological stress may be regarded as a *cause* of MTLP in those women whose emotional and mental status causes them to be malnourished. Indeed, I have observed clinically a number of such cases. However, MTLP will not develop in a woman who takes into her body all the essential elements of nutrition for her particular pregnancy regardless of her psychic disturbance. This implies normal liver function. Hypertension may result from emotional stress, but this is not the hypertension of MTLP. (See Chapter 2.)

TOXEMIA IS RELATED TO ATMOSPHERIC, TELLURIC CONDITIONS

In "modern times" it is difficult to imagine why anyone would want to seriously consider that "atmospheric conditions" could in any way *cause* a severe metabolic disease. It is my hope that this book will help free the minds of certain academic obstetricians from this and many similar fruitless speculations.

CHAPTER 11

IMPLICATIONS FOR PREVENTIVE MEDICINE AND PUBLIC HEALTH

IN CERTAIN AREAS of our nation the incidence of pregnancy complications and neonatal morbidity and mortality are rising. Among Negro women delivering their first pregnancies at the University Hospital, Jackson, Mississippi, 35 per cent are experiencing metabolic toxemia of late pregnancy.[49] At Jefferson Davis Hospital, Houston, Texas, the percentage of women having prenatal care has been falling steadily for the past several years, while the incidence of pregnancy anemias, abruptions of the placenta and toxemia is rising.[73] Only 50 per cent of the women who deliver in city-county hospitals in New York City have any prenatal care. These facts reflect deep-rooted socioeconomic problems, poverty and lack of education. It seems inescapable that if we wish to make available the fruits of modern obstetrical science to all our pregnant women and if we wish to give all the infants born in this nation an equal chance for survival and a decent life with an intact central nervous system, then we must improve the prenatal care and the prenatal nutrition of large numbers of American women of all races.

With the correct orientation toward pregnancy nutrition as presented in this book, it should be possible for public health authorities to introduce widely an aggressive and effective program of public education about the health needs of the pregnant woman. It is possible for a pregnant woman to have a quart of skim milk and two eggs daily, the protein foundation of good pregnancy nutrition, for less than the cost of a pack of cigarettes.

Public health nurses with the correct orientation toward pregnancy nutrition will be so much more effective in their educational and guidance work among women in our lowest class. These public health nurses thus can play a vital role in improving the lives of millions of our American people. I have great faith in the American people, in their ingenuity and ability to organize to solve human problems once they can grasp the correct and scientific views of these problems. This is our great American heritage and we must be true to it.

CHAPTER 12

QUESTIONS FOR FUTURE RESEARCH

In 1865 CLAUDE BERNARD wrote:

> In medicine, we are often confronted with poorly observed and indefinite facts which form actual obstacles in science, in that men always bring them up, saying: it is a fact, it must be accepted. Rational science based on a necessary determinism, must never repudiate an accurate and well-observed fact; but on the same principle, it ought not to encumber itself with apparent facts collected without precision, and possessing no kind of meaning, which are used as a double-edge weapon to support or disprove the most diverse opinions.
>
> In short, science rejects the indeterminate; and in medicine, when we begin to base our opinions on medical tact, on inspiration, or on more or less vague intuition about things, we are outside science and offer an example of that fanciful medicine which may involve the greatest dangers, by surrendering the health and life of the sick to an inspired ignoramus.
>
> True science teaches us to doubt, and, in ignorance, to refrain.[76]

I am closing this book with many unanswered questions. However, I believe my work, if not immediately, in time, will pave the way for rapid and sure progress in answering these questions. I have been able to establish a certain scientific foundation for more detailed biochemical understanding of this problem. I am by training and inclination a clinician and not a biochemist. One motivation in writing this book is to show clearly how this disease can be prevented with our present knowledge. Another motivation is to sweep away those theories which I consider are holding back scientific progress in this field. Another motivation is to attempt to correct some of the irrational clinical practices which have become established in obstetrics regarding prenatal nutrition, practices which I have observed to cause harm to both pregnant women and their babies.

Here are some of the unanswered questions for future investigations.

1. What is the exact nature of the malnutrition which causes MTLP? Protein deficiency? Deficiency of one or more of the essential amino acids? What is the role, if any, of dietary fat? Is there an associated vitamin deficiency? Is there a relatively simple biochemical test to aid in the differential diagnosis in women with the signs and symptoms of this disease?
2. What is the exact role of the gastrointestinal bacteria?
3. What damages the endothelial cells in the liver, kidneys, lungs, adrenals, etc.?
4. What causes convulsions? What causes hypertension?
5. What role do steroids play in the salt and water retention?
6. What is the cause of the hypoalbuminemia?
7. Why do some women have toxemic convulsions when they are "dry"? When they have normal blood pressures?
8. What is the relationship between the "toxemia syndrome" occasionally encountered in molar pregnancy and metabolic toxemia of late pregnancy? Do they share some mechanisms in common? Are molar pregnancies also caused by malnutrition?

It is my hope that most of these questions can be answered in experimental animals and not in pregnant women, for we should rapidly eliminate this sometimes lethal disease now that we can grasp its basic cause: *malnutrition.*

BIBLIOGRAPHY

CHAPTER 1—INTRODUCTION

1. BERNARD, CLAUDE: *An Introduction to the Study of Experimental Medicine (1865).* New York, Colliers, 1961.

CHAPTER 2—CLINICAL DEFINITION AND DIFFERENTIAL DIAGNOSIS

2. BREWER, THOMAS H.: Metabolic toxemia of late pregnancy: definition and differential diagnosis. *Ob/Gyn Digest* (in press).
3. POEN, HAN TJIWAN, AND DJODJO PRANTO, MOELJONE: The possible etiologic factors in hydatidiform mole and choriocarcinoma. *Amer. J. Obstet. Gynec.,* 92:510, 1965.

CHAPTER 3—PATHOLOGY

4. ACOSTA-SISON, H.: A clinicopathologic study of eclampsia based on thirty-eight autopsied cases. *Amer. J. Obstet. Gynec.,* 22:35, 1936.
5. MAQUEO, MANUEL, AYALA, LUIS, AND CERVANTES, LUIS: Nutritional status and liver function in toxemia of pregnancy. *Obstet. Gynec.,* 23:222, 1964.
6. CALL, M. AND LORENTZEN, D.: Rupture of the liver associated with toxemia. *Obstet. Gynec.,* 25:466, 1965.

CHAPTER 4—ABNORMAL PHYSIOLOGY AND BIOCHEMISTRY

Hypovolemia, Hemoconcentration, Hypoalbuminemia

7. DIECKMANN, W.J.: *The Toxemias of Pregnancy,* 2nd ed., St. Louis, Mosby, 1952.
8. STRAUSS, M.B.: Observations on the etiology of toxemias of pregnancy. *Amer. J. Med. Sci., 190:811,* 1935.
9. MACK, H.C.: *The Plasma Proteins in Pregnancy,* Springfield, Ill., Thomas, 1955.
10. LAGERCRANTZ, C.: Electrophoretic analysis of serum in pregnancy and pregnancy toxemia. *Acta Soc. Med. Upsal., 51:117,* 1945.
11. BREWER, THOMAS H.: Limitations of diuretic therapy in the management of severe toxemia: the significance of hypoalbuminemia. *Amer. J. Obstet. Gynec., 83:1352,* 1962.
12. BREWER, THOMAS H.: Administration of human serum albumin in severe toxaemia of pregnancy. *J. Obstet. Gynaec. Brit. Comm., 70:1001,* 1963.

13. STEINFELD, JESSE L.: Differences in daily albumin synthesis between normal men and women as measured with I_{131}-labeled albumin, *J. Lab. Clin. Med.*, *55*:904, 1960.

14. LONGSWORTH, LEWIS G., CURTIS, RAYMOND M., AND PEMBROKE, RICHARD H., JR.: The electrophoretic analysis of maternal and fetal plasmas and sera. *J. Clin. Invest.*, *24*:46, 1945.

15. BUCKINGHAM, JOHN C., McELVIN, THOMAS W., BOWERS, VICTOR M., AND McVAG, JOHN: A clinical study of hydramnios. *Obstet. Gynec.*, *15*:652, 1960.

16. SATO, SHIOICHI: *Pathophysiology of Toxemia of Late Pregnancy.* Tokyo, Igaku Shoin, 1964.

Hepatic Dysfunction

17. BENGTSSON, LARS PH., AND EJARQUE, PETER M.: Production rate of progesterone in the last month of pregnancy. *Acta Obstet. Gynec. Scand.*, *43*:49, 1964.

18. FRUTON, JOSEPH S., AND SIMMONDS, SOFIA: *General Biochemistry,* 2nd ed., New York, Wiley & Sons, 1959, pp. 537 and 646.

19. VENNING, ELEANOR: Endocrine aspects of toxemia. *Clin. Obstet. Gynec.*, *1*:359, 1958.

20. SHEARMAN, RODNEY P.: Some aspects of urinary excretion of pregnanediol in pregnancy. *J. Obstet. Gynaec. Brit. Comm.*, *66*:1, 1959.

21. KUMAR, D., AND BARNES, ALLAN C.: Aldosterone in normal and abnormal pregnancy. *Obstet. Gynec. Survey*, *15*:625, 1960.

22. FRANTZ, ANDREW G., KATZ, FRED H., AND JAILER, JOSEPH W.: 6-Beta-hydroxy-cortisol: high levels in human urine in pregnancy and toxemia. *Proc. Soc. Exp. Biol. Med.*, *105*:41, 1960.

23. ETON, BRUCE, AND SHORT, R.V.: Blood progesterone levels in abnormal pregnancies. *J. Obstet. Gynaec. Brit. Comm.*, *67*:785, 1960.

24. PARKER, FREDERIC, JR., AND TENNEY, BENJAMIN: A study of estrogenic content of the tissues in pregnancy. *Endocrinology*, *23*:492, 1938.

25. RUMBOLZ, WILLIAM L.: The small full-term infant and placental insufficiency. *Western J. Surg.*, *69*:53, 1961.

26. BREWER, THOMAS H., AND HJELTE, VIRGINIA: Bromosulfophthalein conjugation in toxemia of late pregnancy. *Amer. J. Obstet. Gynec.*, *92*:1114, 1965.

27. BREWER, THOMAS H.: Role of malnutrition, hepatic dysfunction and gastro-intestinal bacteria in the pathogenesis of acute toxemia of pregnancy. *Amer. J. Obstet. Gynec.*, *84*:1253, 1962.

28. KRUPP, PHILIP, AND KRUPP, IRIS: Serotonin and toxemia of pregnancy. *Obstet. Gynec., 15*:237, 1960.
29. BREWER, T.H., AND MIALE, J.B.: Glucuronic acid conjugation of anisic acid in normal and toxemic pregnancy. *Obstet Gynec., 20*: 345, 1962.
30. WHIPPLE, GEORGE H.: *The Dynamic Equilibrium of Body Proteins: Hemoglobin, Plasma Proteins, Organ and Tissue Proteins,* Springfield, Ill., Thomas, 1955.
31. KRAUSS, VON ANNELIESE: Blutammoniak bei Schwangesheftgestosen. *Zbl. Gynaek., 83*:2024, 1961.

"Rat Eclampsia"

32. HIMSWORTH, H.P., AND GLYNN, L.E.: Massive hepatic necrosis and diffuse hepatic fibrosis (acute yellow atrophy and portal cirrhosis): their production by means of diet. *Clin. Sci., 5*:93, 1944.
33. GYORGY, P., AND GOLDBLATT, H.: Further observations on the production and prevention of dietary hepatic injury in rats. *J. Exp. Med., 89*:245, 1949.
34. MCKAY, DONALD: The placenta in experimental toxemia. *Obstet. Gynec., 20*:1, 1962.
35. HIBBARD, BRYAN M.: The role of folic acid in pregnancy with particular reference to anemia, abruption and abortion. *J. Obstet. Gynaec. Brit. Comm., 71*:529, 1964.

Toxic Abruptio Placentae: A Theory of Pathogenesis

36. RAMSEY, ELIZABETH M., CORNER, GEORGE W., JR., AND DONNER, MARTIN W.: Serial and cineradiographic visualization of maternal circulation in the primate (hemochorial) placenta. *Amer. J. Obstet. Gynec., 86*:213, 1963.
37. PRITCHARD, J.A. AND WRIGHT, M.R.: Pathogenesis of hypofibrinogenemia in placental abruption. *New Eng. J. Med., 261*:218, 1959.

Renal Dysfunction

38. BURWELL, C.S.: The placenta as a modified arteriovenous fistula in relation to the circulatory adjustments of pregnancy. *Amer. J. Med. Sci., 195*:1, 1938.

How Delivery of the Placenta and Fetus Improves the Clinical Condition of the Toxemic Patient

39. DEXTER, LEWIS, AND WEISS, SOMA: *Preeclamptic and Eclamptic Toxemias of Pregnancy,* Boston, Little, Brown, 1941.

CHAPTER 6—OBESITY, WEIGHT GAIN, DIETARY SALT AND DIURETICS: A PERSPECTIVE

40. JACOBSON, H.N., BURKE, B.S., SMITH, C.A., AND REID, D.E.: Effect of weight reduction in obese pregnant women in pregnancy, labor and delivery and on the condition of the infant at birth. *Amer. J. Obstet. Gynec., 83*:1609, 1962.

41. SAND, RICHARD X.: Obesity and pregnancy. *Amer. J. Obstet. Gynec., 83*:1617, 1962.

42. PEDLOW, P.R.B.: The significance of weight gains and losses during selected periods of pregnancy in Jamaican women. *J. Obstet. Gynaec. Brit. Comm., 71*:908, 1964.

43 ROBINSON, MARGARET: Salt in pregnancy. *Lancet, 1*:178 (Jan. 25), 1958.

44. MENGERT, W.F., AND TACCHI, D.A.: Pregnancy toxemia and sodium chloride. *Amer. J. Obstet. Gynec., 81*:601, 1961.

45. BOWER, DAVID: The influence of dietary salt intake on pre-eclampsia. *J. Obstet. Gynaec. Brit. Comm., 71*:123, 1964.

46. FLOWERS, CHARLES E., GRIZZLE, JAMES E., EASTERLY, WILLIAM E., AND BONNER, O. BLANCHARD: Chlorothiazide as a prophylaxis against toxemia of pregnancy. *Amer. J. Obstet. Gynec., 84*:919, 1962.

(See also refs. 11 and 12 above.)

CHAPTER 7—PRINCIPLES OF MANAGEMENT

47. MENGERT, W.F., AND TWEEDIE, JAMES A.: Acute vasospastic toxemia: therapeutic nihilism. *Obstet. Gynec., 24*:662, 1964.

(See also ref. 12 above.)

CHAPTER 8—PREVENTION THROUGH PRENATAL NUTRITIONAL EDUCATION

48. HAMLIN, R.H.J.: Prophylaxis against toxemia. *Clin. Obstet. Gynec., 1*:369, 1958.

49. NEWTON, MICHAEL: The continuing problem of eclampsia. *Surg. Gynec. Obstet., 118*:1055, 1964.

CHAPTER 9—"HIGH RISK" PATIENTS

The Teen-age Mother-to-be

50. MUSSIO, THOMAS J.: Primigravidas under age 14. *Amer. J. Obstet. Gynec., 84*:442, 1962.

51. WALLACE, HELEN: Teen-age pregnancy. *Amer. J. Obstet. Gynec., 92*;1125, 1965.

The "Unwed Mother"

52. DODEK, SAMUEL M.: Personal communication, Washington, D.C., 1960.

Women in Poverty

53. NELSON, ROBERT L., AND BREWER, THOMAS H.: Toxemia of pregnancy at Jackson Memorial Hospital. *Bull. Univ. Miami Sch. Med., 12*:87, 1958.

54. MAYER, JEAN: Food habits and nutritional status of American Negroes. *Postgrad. Med., 37*:A-110, 1965.

Twin Gestation: Eating for Three

55. FARRELL, A.G.W.: Twin pregnancy. A study of 1000 cases. *S. Afr. J. Obstet. Gynaec., 2*:35, 1964.

Food Habits, Fads and Foolish Notions

56. FERGUSON, J.H., AND KEATON, A.G.: Studies of diets of pregnant women in Mississippi: ingestion of clay and laundry starch. *New Orleans Med. Sci. J., 102*:460, 1950.

Diabetes Mellitus

57. PEEL, JOHN: Progress in knowledge and management of the pregnant diabetic patient. *Amer. J. Obstet. Gynec., 83*:847, 1962.

Medical Problems

58. TENNEY, BENJAMIN, AND DANDROW, ROBERT V.: Clinical study of hypertensive disease in pregnancy. *Amer. J. Obstet. Gynec., 81*:8, 1961.

59. RAURAMO, LAURI: Fertility, pregnancy and labor in women with a history of nephritis or pyelonephritis. *Acta Obstet. Gynec. Scand., 41*:357, 1962.

60. DRAA, C.C.: Personal communication, Chicago, 1957.

CHAPTER 10—"RED HERRINGS" IN "TOXEMIA" RESEARCH

61. PAGE, ERNEST W.: The relation between hydatid moles, relative ischemia of the gravid uterus and the placental origin of eclampsia. *Amer. J. Obstet. Gynec., 37*:291, 1939.

62. OGDEN, E., HILDEBRAND, G.J., AND PAGE, E.W.: Rise of blood pressure during ischemia of the gravid uterus. *Proc. Soc. Exp. Biol. Med., 43*:49, 1940.

63. KUMAR, D.: Chronic placental ischemia in relation to toxemias of pregnancy. *Amer. J. Obstet. Gynec., 84*:1323, 1962.

64. HUNTER, C.A., AND HOWARD, W.F.: A pressor substance (hystero-

tonin) occurring in toxemia. *Amer. J. Obstet. Gynec., 79*:838, 1960.

65. BREWER, TOM: Toxemia of pregnancy. *Amer. J. Obstet. Gynec., 89*:838, 1964. (This is a refutation of the utero-placental ischemia theory of the pathogenesis of metabolic toxemia of late pregnancy.)

66. NORTON, EDWARD, W.D.: Personal communication, Miami, 1962.

67. KEARNS, THOMAS: Opthalmoscopic findings in pregnant diabetic patients. *Clin. Obstet. Gynec., 5*:379, 1962.

68. TRAUT, H.F., AND KUDER, A.: The lesions in 1,500 placentas considered from a clinical point of view. *Amer. J. Obstet. Gynec., 27*: 552, 1934.

69. SOPHIAN, JOHN: Myometrial resistance to stretch the cause of pre-eclampsia. *J. Obstet. Gynec. Brit. Comm., 62*:37, 1955.

70. BEACHAM, WOODARD D., HERNQUIST, WILLIAM C., BEACHAM, DAN W., AND WEBSTER, HERMAN D.: Abdominal pregnancy at Charity in New Orleans. *Amer. J. Obstet. Gynec., 84*:1257, 1962.

71. BENJAMIN, FRED, AND CRAIG, C.J.T.: Uterine distention and pre-eclamptic toxaemia. *J. Obstet. Gynaec. Brit. Comm., 68*:827, 1961.

72. BREWER, T.H.: Abstract #1093. *Excerpta Med. [X], 18*:232, 1965. (This is an abstract of ref. 12 above with a refutation of the utero-renal reflex theory of pathogenesis of metabolic toxemia of late pregnancy. It also contains a theory of the pathogenesis of hydramnios associated with toxemia.)

CHAPTER 11—IMPLICATIONS FOR PREVENTIVE MEDICINE AND PUBLIC HEALTH

73. JOHNSTON, ROBERT A., FRANKLIN, ROBERT, AND ROFFMAN, LARRY: Is prenatal care beneficial or necessary? *Southern Med. J., 57*:399, 1964.

(see also excellent discussion of this article in *Obstet. Gynec. Survey, 19*:741, 1964.)

74. BURKE, BERTHA S., BEAL, VIRGINIA A., KIRKWOOD, SAMUEL B., AND STUART, HAROLD C.: Nutritional studies during pregnancy. *Amer. J. Obstet. Gynec., 46*:38, 1943.

75. JARVINEN, P.A. AND TARJONNE, H.: Observations on the value of prenatal care on maternal mortality and eclampsia of pregnancy. *Ann. Chir. Gynaec. Fenn., 53*:91, 1964.

CHAPTER 12—QUESTIONS FOR FUTURE RESEARCH

76. BERNARD, CLAUDE, *op. cit.*

INDEX

APPENDIX TO THIS NEW EDITION

CHAPTER 13

APPENDIX TO THIS NEW EDITION

I. *Pregnant? . . . and want a healthy child*

From 1963 to 1969 I used no printed materials in my prenatal care-nutrition education program in Contra Costa County, California. I depended on personal communications via group lecture-discussions with the pregnant ladies as a routine part of their first prenatal visit to our clinics and then on constant follow-up discussions about their diets with each patient *at every return prenatal care visit.* This is what Mrs. Agnes Higgins of the Montreal Diet Dispensary refers to as "eyeball to eyeball counseling." It soon became clear to each pregnant patient that her "doctor" (me) considered her diet as the highest priority item in maintaining her health and the health, growth and development of her unborn baby. Furthermore, I actually practiced throughout the entire gestation the basic principles I had set forth at the first visit.

At the end of 1969 in an effort to move these methods out into the world and to stimulate thinking and discussion in this area of nutrition/malnutrition in human pregnancy, I wrote a booklet to take to President Nixon's White House "Hunger Conference" held in the first week of December, 1969, in Washington, D.C.: *PREGNANT? . . . and want a healthy child.* Excerpts from this booklet appear below including a written representation of the basic diet plan. (The "alternative combinations" for vegetarians were added after I left the clinics in 1976.) Information in this form has been distributed with over 200,000 booklets and leaflets in the last twelve years. I know of no single instance where this information has caused harm to a mother or a baby. (I began to hand this out to my clinic patients in November, 1969.)

PREGNANT? . . . and want a healthy child

by TOM BREWER, M.D., Author:
Metabolic Toxemia of Late Pregnancy: A Disease of Malnutrition

The Importance of Diet

If you are an expectant mother, you must eat a good, nutritious, balanced diet *every day* during your pregnancy. A good diet is the best insurance that your baby will be healthy and strong, with a normal weight at birth!

The Dangers of Bad Diet

Forty years of medical research has proved that bad diets during pregnancy cause:
1. Stillborn babies.
2. Low birth weight or premature babies.
3. Brain-damaged babies with less intelligence.
4. Hyperactive babies with more irritability.
5. Infection-prone babies with more illness.

A good diet will protect your baby from these troubles.
Bad diets cause diseases in mothers, too:
1. Metabolic Toxemia of Late Pregnancy (MTLP)—a disease caused by too little high quality proteins and vitamins in the diet. Women with MTLP suffer convulsions or "fits," coma, heart failure, fat in their livers, bleeding into their livers and often death for both mother and baby. It is estimated that in the United States 30,000 babies die each year of MTLP—and thousands more live with damage to their brains. They suffer cerebral palsy, epilepsy and other nervous system disorders.

A good diet will protect you and your baby from MTLP.
2. Anemias ("low blood")—caused by not enough iron, vitamins and/or protein in the diet.

A good diet will protect you from anemias.
3. Abruption of the Placenta or "Afterbirth"—a disease in which the afterbirth tears loose inside the mother's womb, often before labor begins; the mother bleeds and the baby dies in 50 per cent of the cases.

A good diet will protect you and your baby from Abruption.
4. Severe infections of the lungs, kidneys and liver.

A good diet will protect you and your baby from severe infections.

5. Miscarriage—if the mother does not have a good diet, the placenta grows imperfectly and cannot meet the needs of the developing baby, so a miscarriage results.

A good diet will protect you and your baby from miscarriages.

What Is a Good, Nutritious, Balanced Diet?

When you are pregnant, you need more of good quality foods than when you are not pregnant. To meet your own needs and those of your developing baby, you must have, *every day*, at least:

1. One quart (four glasses) of milk—any kind: whole milk, low fat, skim, powdered skim or buttermilk. If you do not like milk, you can substitute one cup of yoghurt for each cup of milk.
2. Two eggs.
3. Two servings of fish, shellfish, chicken or turkey, lean beef, veal, lamb, pork, liver or kidney.

Alternative combinations include:
Rice with: beans, cheese, sesame, milk
Cornmeal with: beans, cheese, tofu, milk
Beans with: rice, bulgar, cornmeal, wheat noodles, sesame seeds, milk
Peanuts with: sunflower seeds, milk
Whole wheat bread or noodles with: beans, cheese, peanut butter, milk, tofu

For each serving of meat, you can substitute these quantities of cheese:

Brick— 4 oz.
Camembert—6 oz.
Cheddar—3 oz.
Cottage—6 oz.
Longhorn—3 oz.
Muenster—4 oz.
Monterey Jack—4 oz.
Swiss—3 oz.

4. Two servings of fresh, green leafy vegetables: mustard, beet, collard, dandelion or turnip greens, spinach, lettuce, cabbage, broccoli, kale, Swiss chard.

5. Five servings of whole grain breads, rolls, cereals or pancakes: wheatena, 100% bran flakes, granola, shredded wheat, wheat germ, oatmeal, buckwheat or whole wheat pancakes, corn bread, corn tortillas, corn or bran or whole wheat muffins, waffles, brown rice.
6. Two choices from: a whole potato (any style), large green pepper, grapefruit, lemon, lime papaya, tomato (one piece of fruit or one large glass juice).
7. Three pats of butter.

Also include in your diet:

8. A yellow or orange-colored vegetable or fruit five times a week.
9. Liver once a week.
10. Table salt: SALT YOUR FOOD TO TASTE.
11. Water: drink to thirst.

It is not healthy for you and your unborn baby to go even 24 hours without good food!

Certain Things May Prevent You from Having a Good Diet

A good diet sounds simple, doesn't it? But it isn't so simple in our society. Many things may happen to prevent you from eating and digesting a good diet each day throughout pregnancy.

You may believe that the foods you see widely advertised on TV and in magazines give you and your baby the proteins, vitamins and minerals you need. Foods such as: boxed cereals, white bread, potato chips, soft drinks, candy, french fries, commercial cakes and cookies provide expensive, useless "empty" calories. When you spend money on these foods, you are not getting your money's worth of good nutrition. The first items to put in your shopping cart are the foods on the good diet list!

Another situation which may interfere with your good diet is the nausea and vomiting, or heartburn, indigestion and loss of appetite which many women experience in pregnancy. This problem must be corrected quickly, with the help of your doctor, so that you can resume your good eating habits.

If you are overweight at the beginning of your pregnancy, you may think that now is a good time to try to lose some of that extra weight. Pregnancy is not the time to go on a low-calorie diet. There is recent evidence that your baby's brain is growing at its most rapid rate during the last two months of pregnancy. Mothers who follow low-calorie diets risk stunting the growth of their babies' brains.

The Doctor May Stand Between You And Good Nutrition

MISINFORMATION ABOUT DIET

You will often meet a doctor, in a private office or in a clinic, who doesn't really understand the life-and-death importance of a good diet for you and your baby.

You may not be told anything about the need for a good diet for you and your baby.

You may be told that diet "isn't too important" for your health or for the health of your unborn child. Don't believe it!

You may be told that salt, ordinary table salt, is harmful to you and your baby. Don't believe it! Continue to salt your food to taste.

MISINFORMATION ABOUT WEIGHT GAIN

You may be told to go on a starvation-type diet if you "gain too much weight." Don't go on a starvation diet! The food you eat every day while you are pregnant builds the bones, muscle and brain of your baby. Pounds gained while you are on a good diet protect and prepare you for labor and breast feeding.

If you gain a few extra pounds during this pregnancy from eating a nutritious, balanced diet, it won't hurt you or the baby—even if you gain fifty or sixty pounds. Worry if you don't gain enough.

MISINFORMATION ABOUT DANGEROUS DRUGS

You may be given "diet pills" to take away your appetite, drugs like Dexidrene or "speed" (amphetamines) . Don't take them!

These drugs are not healthy for you. They are not healthy for your unborn baby. Who would give a baby "speed"? Every drug you take passes quickly into the placenta or afterbirth, then into the baby's bloodstream and body.

The amphetamines are given to kill the hungry mother's appetite. They also give her an unnatural boost. They relieve depression, make her feel she is working smoother and living a healthful life—even though she is not getting enough to eat. In this way, amphetamines cover up her problem of poor nutrition.

You may be given diuretics or "water pills" during your pregnancy. The immediate effect of these pills is to cause your body to eliminate water excessively. They dry you up. They dry up your baby. Don't take them!

These drugs are *not* needed to have a healthy pregnancy and a healthy baby, however, the private drug industry has widely promoted diuretics and amphetamines for use in mothers. These "hard sell" promotions, along with the low calorie, low salt diet and indifference of many doctors toward pregnancy nutrition, have created a grave health hazard for American women and their unborn children.

Water pills have damaged many pregnant women and their babies. Reported bad effects listed by the drug companies who, nevertheless, continued to advertise them, include:

1. Loss of appetite
2. Stomach irritation
3. Nausea and vomiting
4. Diarrhea
5. Constipation
6. Cramping
7. Muscle spasm
8. Jaundice
9. Pancreatitis
10. Hyperglycemia
11. High blood pressure
12. Dizziness
13. Headache
14. Thrombocytopenia
15. Glycosuria
16. Aplastic anemia
17. Skin rash
18. Weakness
19. Restlessness
20. Photosensitivity

The doctor often prescribes these drugs to "treat" the *normal* swelling that occurs during pregnancy! If you have been eating a good, well-balanced, nutritious diet, you will probably have swelling of your feet, hands and face—normally.

If the swelling bothers you, lie down a few minutes with your feet elevated. You can repeat this simple remedy several times a day if needed.

Remember: it is not healthy for you and your unborn baby to go even 24 hours without good food!

AFTERWORD TO THIS EDITION BY THE AUTHOR

FIFTEEN YEARS have passed since this work was first published. During this time many studies have been done which strongly support its basic nutritional thesis and clinical obstetrical practices. I have also "discovered" many studies in this same line from the 1930s, 1940s, 1950s which have been buried by Western obstetrics for decades. In the Appendix an annotated bibliography of scientific studies is presented which focuses on those works which form the foundation of a modern methodology of primary prevention of human pregnancy pathology, diseases and deaths of both mothers and their unborn and newborn babies.

In the United States in 1982 officially the cause of metabolic toxemia of late pregnancy (MTLP) remains entirely "unknown." This is unfortunate because primary prevention of this disease entity can not be carried out in human prenatal care with any scientific certainty by nutritionally ignorant physicians. Tragic cases of MTLP continue to be brought to our attention nearly every week now from all over the United States.

THE COMPLETE SCARSDALE
MEDICAL DIET IN PREGNANCY

A few weeks before his death, I had a discussion with Herman Tarnower, M.D., about a mother who died in Washington, D.C., on August 16, 1979, during her second pregnancy. Mrs. F.C.A., age 31, from early in her fatal pregnancy had followed Dr. Tarnower's "Complete Scarsdale Medical Diet" and restricted her dietary salt intake for blind weight control. This diet afforded her less than 1,000 calories daily, a low salt intake and directly caused intrauterine fetal growth retardation and MTLP. Shocked, Tarnower agreed to put a more explicit warning about the dangers of such severe calorie and salt restriction during pregnancy in the next edition of his popular book. He had believed that

MTLP was caused by *excessive* salt and calories in the diet.

One month after her death from MTLP I was able to obtain a three-hour interview with this woman's husband, a college graduate and articulate historian. The errors and neglect in her traditional, non-nutritional, AMA style "prenatal care" are so glaring and tragic that they should be recorded for everyone to read, so they can be stopped for all women!

Mrs. F.C.A. had had a normal first pregnancy and birth 14 months before her death from MTLP in her second pregnancy. At the start of her first pregnancy she had weighed 120 pounds and was 5 feet, 4 inches in height. She ate well and gained 35 pounds, to 155. She and her husband had prepared childbirth (Lamaze) classes; she took no drugs during pregnancy, labor or delivery and had a "natural childbirth." Her normal baby boy weighed 6 pounds, 15 ounces and was 20 inches in length. She had no complications and breast fed the baby for seven months until she became pregnant again.

At the beginning of her second pregnancy Mrs. F.C.A. weighed 135 pounds (height still 5'4") and she felt "panic" at the idea of gaining another 35 pounds during pregnancy: "135 plus 35 equals 170" she thought. Thus she decided to go on the "Complete Scarsdale Medical Diet" of less than 1,000 calories daily and to restrict dietary salt. She received permission from her obstetrician to follow this diet. From time to time her husband went on the diet with her; neither had the slightest fear of malnutrition during pregnancy.

She gained no weight during the first six months of this second pregnancy. After three weeks on the diet she began to feel tired, weak, and found it increasingly difficult to look after her baby. In a few more weeks she lost her appetite, felt nauseated and "miserable," yet she was proud of the fact that she was gaining no weight. Between the sixth month and seventh month prenatal visits to her obstetrician, she gained nine pounds. Her face, hands and feet began to swell; she had headaches. She began to have abdominal pains. A few days before her last prenatal appointment she went to a jeweler to have the rings cut off her fingers.

On this last visit her blood pressure was "normal." She was swollen up, had gained 9 pounds of water in a month while starving herself, had pain in her right upper abdomen, was tired, weak, nauseated, had headaches; yet her doctor remained oblivious to her peril and sent her home with the customary "Everything is going to be all right, dear."

That same night her abdominal pain became more severe, and at 5:00 A.M. the next morning she was admitted to the hospital as a possible gall bladder attack. Her blood pressure was now elevated but this was attributed to her pain. She was given morphine for pain. A general surgeon was called and ordered an X-ray of her abdomen. She had an eclamptic seizure while on the X-ray table in the hospital. It was only then that the diagnosis of "eclampsia" was made! She was given a battery of drugs including furosemide (Lasix®-Hoechst), a most potent salt diuretic contraindicated in pregnancy. A few hours later the fetal heart stopped. A Cesarean section was done with delivery of a 2 pound, 9 ounce stillborn. She went into shock and suffered irreversible brain damage. She was kept alive on a respirator for a week and then, since repeated brain wave tracings were "flat" signifying "brain death," the machine was turned off and she was allowed to die.

Many different physicians attended Mrs. F.C.A. during her terminal illness; these included her obstetrician, a general surgeon, an internist, a radiologist, a neurologist, a neurosurgeon, an opthalmologist (eye specialist), a hematologist (blood specialist), a neonatologist (newborn disease specialist), and several different residents. They all told her husband that the cause of her disease, "eclampsia," is unknown, that there is no known method of prevention of this "mysterious disease." Not one of these doctors took a detailed medical history as is recorded here; not one asked the still forbidden question in USA obstetrics: *"What had she been eating?"* This question, if asked earlier in this pregnancy, could have saved her life and the life of her unborn baby in 1979.

(Note: After her death, her husband found in her purse at home the urine specimen which she had taken to her last prenatal visit with her obstetrician; she had obviously forgotten to turn it in for analysis.)

THE LOW CALORIE, LOW SALT, HIGH WATER DIET IN PREGNANCY

Mrs. N.L.L., age 29, was a school teacher in a midwestern city. She had a master's degree from college; her husband is a Ph.D. chemist employed by a large chemical corporation. They had postponed pregnancy for several years during his postgraduate education. They attended prepared childbirth classes (Lamaze) and she had traditional, AMA style prenatal care. At 32 weeks gestation she was observed to have some swelling of her feet and ankles and had gained 25 pounds which her obstetrician considered the upper limit for her. Height was five feet two inches and pre-pregnancy weight was 145 pounds. Her doctor gave her a low calorie, low salt diet to follow and advised that she drink at least eight large glasses of water daily.

Thus in early March, 1981, *she taped the low calorie, low salt diet to her refrigerator door and carefully followed it for the next five weeks.* She forced down the extra water with considerable difficulty. In spite of her rigid compliance with her doctor's orders, Mrs. N.L.L. developed MTLP in the 35th week of gestation and by the 37th week had an eclamptic convulsion in the hospital. A Cesarean section was done an hour after her first convulsion; blood loss was described as "excessive." Twelve hours after surgery she collapsed in shock with pulmonary edema. Like Mrs. F.C.A., she suffered brain death and was kept alive for two days on a respirator. On April 13, 1981 with the consent of her family the machine was turned off and she was allowed to die. Her five pound, six ounce baby boy survived, motherless.

THE LOW CALORIE, LOW SALT DIET AND SODIUM DIURETICS IN PREGNANCY

Janine Ricozzi, age 28, died of MTLP ("eclampsia") on March 10, 1977, in Westchester County, New York. It was her first pregnancy. She never missed a prenatal visit with her obstetrician who is highly respected in his field. Mrs. Ricozzi followed her doctor's advice meticulously, as she had been trying for six years to become pregnant.

Early in pregnancy Janine was told not to gain over "two

pounds a month" or a total of 18 pounds. Her pre-pregnancy weight was 130 pounds and her height was five feet, two inches. On February 2, 1977, at about 24-weeks gestation her doctor gave her a prescription for Abbott's thiazide diuretic, Enduron®, and told her to ingest no dietary salt because she had developed some swelling of her feet and ankles. On the low calorie, low salt diet and diuretic her swelling gradually increased to include her face and hands and she became tired and weak. She developed nausea, vomiting, abdominal pain which her doctor diagnosed over the telephone as the "flu" on February 28; three hours later she had her first eclamptic convulsion at home and was rushed to the hospital where her obstetrician was initially reluctant to make the diagnosis of eclampsia until she was observed to have another grand mal seizure in the hospital emergency room. She began to receive a battery of drugs intravenously including Valium®, magnesium sulfate, hydralazine and furosemide (Lasix®-Hoechst), a most potent sodium diuretic contraindicated in pregnancy. In fact, during the first 24 hours after admission to the hospital, she was given 200 mgm of Lasix® intravenously, 180 mgm of it administered when she was in shock.

Her blood pressure was 150/100 on admission to the hospital and ranged up to 180/110. Laboratory tests revealed 3-plus proteinuria, serum uric acid over 12 mgm%, hemoglobin 14.9 gm.% and a hematocrit of 45. (Hemoconcentration in malnourished, hypovolemic toxemic women has long been observed to be a grave prognostic sign in this disease.)

The next morning after massive drug therapy had failed and four hours of oxytocin had not been successful in starting labor, she was delivered of a 2 pound, 5 ounce boy at 28-weeks gestation by Cesarean section. Immediately after surgery she became hypotensive and oliguric; four hours later her blood pressure was only 70/50, at which time she was given 80 mgm. of Lasix®. Twenty minutes after the injection of Lasix® she went into profound shock with no blood pressure or carotid pulse; she was apneic for five minutes then blood pressure increased to 70/50 and stayed in the 50/30 to 70/50 range for seven hours when it rose to 100/72. At this time she was given 80 mgm of Lasix® and within 25 minutes her pressure was down to 78/54. During this time an EEG showed no evidence of cerebral activity; she had suffered brain death. She was kept alive on a respirator in the hospital intensive care unit for the next nine days. She remained edematous, never regaining consciousness, with fixed, unresponsive pupils. With the family's consent the respirator was turned off and she was allowed to die on March 10.

Janine Ricozzi had been seriously trying to limit her weight gain to two pounds per month since early pregnancy. For over two months she had been restricting salt and had taken Abbott's thiazide diuretic, Enduron®, from February 2 to February 28 when she had a convulsion, was admitted to the hospital and treated with even more dangerous drugs. After her brain death she had been kept alive in the intensive care unit receiving only intravenous glucose and water for ten days.

The pathologist who did an autopsy on Janine Ricozzi's body began his report:

"Well-developed, well-nourished 28-year-old white female . . ."

MTLP NO LONGER A DISEASE OF POVERTY

These three tragic cases illustrate the fact that MTLP is not a disease limited to women in poverty or to those "without prenatal care" as I thought in 1966. Any woman who suffers malnutrition can develop the disease at any age or parity. In the first case above, Mrs. F.C.A., the malnutrition was so obvious by medical history alone but her doctors did not take such a history. Her obstetrician told her husband:

"Your wife is a strange, unusual case. We usually see eclampsia among the poor, black, unmarried, teenagers, those women without prenatal care, who come into the D.C. General hospital."

This was little consolation to the bereaved husband since his wife was age 31, white, married, was in her second pregnancy, and had traditional, AMA style prenatal care with an OB-GYN specialist.

The type of "prenatal care" which evolved in the United States during the 1950s totally excluded any serious concern for the problems of malnutrition during pregnancy which was simply denied out of existence—and still is in 1982. As a result of this profound nutritional ignorance and nonchalance on the part of the medical profession, the drug industry was able to launch an aggressive promotion for their sodium diuretics and low calorie, low sodium diet sheets which were spread across the nation and the world during the 1960s and 1970s. During this time it has been estimated that over two million pregnancies in the United States each year were subjected to this sort of iatrogenic (doctor-caused) malnutrition with sodium diuretics!

NATIONAL INSTITUTES OF HEALTH IN CONTRA COSTA COUNTY, CALIFORNIA

For twelve and a half years, July 1, 1963 to January 21, 1976, I was able to carry on the prenatal care-nutrition education program first described in this book in 1966. During this time period in our county health services over 7,000 pregnancies were managed with my methodology and there was no single case of convulsive MTLP ("eclampsia"). There was no maternal death. Good nutrition without drugs made pregnant women healthy and produced larger newborns with less prematurity and low birth weight. I was able to see the results with my own eyes. It was obvious that blind fear of weight gain, edema, hypertension in pregnancy had to be abandoned if maternal-fetal health were to be safeguarded in a scientific and humane fashion here in the United States. The traditional assumption that every pregnant woman within the borders of the USA is adequately nourished had to be challenged; iatrogenic malnutrition had to be exposed. Applied nutrition science and physiology had to be brought into human prenatal care as a routine, respectable part of that care for every pregnant woman all through gestation.

In an effort to focus some national attention on this point of view I made repeated efforts after 1966 to interest people in the National Institutes of Health (NIH) in this line of clinical research and practice. From 1971 through 1973 Charles Stark, M.D., Ph.D., and Frank Lundin, M.D., Ph.D., working as epidemiologists for the National Institute of Child Health and Human Development (NICHD) did in fact carry out an independent, retrospective study of 5,615 pregnancies associated with my prenatal care-nutrition education program which were delivered in the Contra Costa County Hospital, Martinez, California, over a five and one-half year period, July 1, 1965 through December 31, 1970. This NIH study was conducted under the direction of Charles U. Lowe, M.D., then Scientific Director of NICHD, who promised me at the beginning a "highly critical, scientific analysis." "We will play the role of the Devil's Advocate," he said to me at the beginning of this study in 1970.

In the *Journal of Reproductive Medicine,* vol. 13, pp. 175, 176, 1974, I made a preliminary report on data given me by the NIH epidemiologists; no other report on this study has ever been published. The Devil's Advocates in the NIH were unable to refute the nutritional thesis of etiology of MTLP just as they were unable to discredit my methods of primary prevention of MTLP with nutrition education and counseling and the abandonment of the low salt, low calorie diet, diuretic, weight limitation regimen in human prenatal care. These NIH data documented the complete eradication of convulsive MTLP and an incidence of milder forms of the disease among high risk, low income women of less than 1.0%.

Among women having their first pregnancies in my prenatal care-nutrition program, 1965-1970, NIH epidemiologists found a more than 10-fold reduction in "pregnancy-induced hypertension (PIH)" when compared with first pregnancies from one of the other Contra Costa County prenatal clinics where the traditional, non-nutritional methods prevailed. ("PIH" was defined by NIH as an observed rise in diastolic blood pressure of 20 mm Hg or more on two occasions at least six hours apart.) Tables A and B present some of the "selected data" from the NIH statistical tables. It is obvious, as in other works, that increasing maternal weight gain is positively correlated with increasing infant birth weight among women trying to eat an adequate diet all through gestation, salting to taste and being protected from harmful drugs. It is also highly significant that the longer the pregnant women were exposed to the nutrition education program as reflected by the number of prenatal visits, the lower the incidence of low birth weight babies and the higher the infant birth weights. In this study no other aspect of the prenatal care could have possibly produced such results except the nutritional status of the women.

It is important to note that these phenomena were observed in all "ethnic groups" created by the NIH epidemiologists: "black" (48%), "white" (42%) and "Spanish surnames" (10%). It is now obvious that "genetics" does not play a major, etiologic role in the ethnic pattern of human reproductive pathology in the United States and throughout the world. Another major myth of racism is thus exposed.

*TABLE A

BIRTH WEIGHT AND MATERNAL WEIGHT GAIN BY "ETHNIC GROUPS"

"Ethnic Group"	*No.*	*Average Wt. Gain Lbs./Week*	*No. Low Birth Wt. (%)*	*Mean Infant Birth Wt. (grams)*
"Black"	36	<0.5	2 (5.6)	3111
	103	0.5 - 0.99	8 (7.8)	3163
	84	1.0 - 1.49	5 (6.0)	3173
	37	≥1.5	1 (2.7)	3574
"White"	21	<0.5	0 (0.0)	3298
	53	0.5 - 0.99	4 (7.5)	3316
	59	1.0 - 1.49	4 (6.8)	3403
	28	≥1.5	0 (0.0)	3679
"Spanish Surname"	7	<0.5	0 (0.0)	3321
	14	0.5 - 0.99	0 (0.0)	3393
	21	1.0 - 1.49	2 (9.5)	3440
	5	≥1.5	0 (0.0)	3643

("Weight gain" is only that recorded from first clinic visit to last weight before delivery. These 468 pregnancies were "selected":" the women were first seen in the Richmond Health Clinic prenatal nutrition program before the end of the 28th week of gestation, for at least 4 visits over a period of 4 or more weeks during pregnancy. These babies were all delivered in the Contra Costa County Hospital, Martinez, California, July 1, 1965 through December 31, 1970.)

* These data were collected and analyzed by epidemiologists of the NICHD-NIH.

*TABLE B

BIRTH WEIGHT AND NUMBER OF
PRENATAL VISITS BY "ETHNIC GROUPS"

"Ethnic Group"	No. Patients	No. Visits	Low Birth Wt. (%)	Mean Birth Wt. (grams)
"Black"	174	1 & 2	30 (17.24)	2977
	369	3 - 9	25 (6.77)	3208
	41	10 & more	0 (0.00)	3311
"White"	190	1 & 2	20 (10.53)	3218
	304	3 - 9	15 (4.93)	3347
	22	10 & more	0 (0.00)	3591
"Spanish	41	1 & 2	3 (7.32)	3323
Surname"	70	3 - 9	2 (2.86)	3357
	9	10 & more	0 (0.00)	3639

(These babies were all born in the Contra Costa County Hospital, Martinez, California, July 1, 1965 through December 31, 1970. These mothers received prenatal care and nutrition education at the Richmond Health Clinic, Richmond, California.)
* These data were collected and analyzed by epidemiologists of the NICHD-NIH.

HYPERTENSION IN PREGNANCY

In the last fifteen years obstetricians have narrowly focused on the blood pressure of the pregnant woman as being of central concern regardless of her nutritional-metabolic status, liver function, blood volume and placental function. If the diastolic blood pressure rises 15 or 20 mm Hg or the systolic rises 20-30 mm Hg, a diagnosis of "pregnancy-induced hypertension" (PIH) is made. All "PIH" is then "managed" the same as if every hypertensive pregnant woman were in jeopardy of convulsions, brain hemorrhage, abruption of the placenta, fetal death, etc. This is simply not true; *most hypertension in human pregnancy is physiological or benign, not related to MTLP at all.*

Without recognizing it, Mathews et al. have shown the benign nature of hypertension in the well-fed pregnant woman. (*British Medical Journal,* vol. 2, p. 623, 1978) When these workers abandoned the traditional "therapies" for hypertension in pregnancy, bed rest, low calorie, low salt diets, sodium diuretics, sedatives, pre-term induction, for women with "non-albuminuric hypertension," they observed the same outcome of pregnancy in such hypertensive women as in normotensive women in their prenatal care clinics. In the United States the outcomes of such hypertensive pregnancies continue to be so poor because of the traditional "therapies," not because the blood pressure rises a few mm Hg.

This differential diagnosis of hypertension in pregnancy is so important and must be brought to the attention of every doctor involved in giving human beings prenatal care:

DIFFERENTIAL DIAGNOSIS OF "HYPERTENSION IN PREGNANCY"

(The accurate diagnosis of hypertension in pregnancy requires a complete medical history, in the patient's own words whenever possible, appropriate lab studies and reflective thought, i.e. differential diagnosis. Rational, scientific clinical management of hypertension in pregnancy can not be accomplished without an accurate clinical diagnosis.)

I. *Physiological (Non-pathologic) Blood Pressure Elevation*
- a) Technical errors in measuring BP: obese arm with narrow cuff, etc.
- b) Rise of BP in 3rd trimester after a physiological fall in the 2nd trimester associated with the placental A-V shunt.
- c) Excitement, emotional stress—temporary, in doctor's office, in labor.
- d) Physical exertion, exercise, active labor.

II. *Metabolic Toxemia of Late Pregnancy (MTLP)*
(A direct result of some type of prenatal malnutrition, i.e. lack of dietary intakes of high biological quality proteins for essential amino acids, calories from carbohydrates, salt (NaCl), water, vitamins, other minerals such as calcium, iron, zinc. Nausea, vomiting, loss of appetite, diarrhea, sodium diuretics often contribute to this malnutrition. Liver dysfunction and maternal *hypovolemia* occur in this disease, sometimes three or four months before the onset of hypertension, edema, proteinuria or other signs of the disease . . . which is entirely preventable now.)

III. *Medical and Surgical Diseases*
   a) Essential hypertension, may first be detected during pregnancy.
   b) Kidney diseases, a long list.
   c) Heart failure.
   d) Coarctation of the aorta.
   e) Pheochromocytoma, adrenal tumor.
   f) Central nervous system disorders: brain tumor, epilepsy, stroke, etc.
   g) Molar pregnancy (may cause severe hypertension in early pregnancy).
IV. *Varying Combinations of I, II, & III above* in the same woman, i.e.
   the woman with chronic essential hypertension may become malnourished, hypovolemic and develop a "superimposed" MTLP. Standard medical "therapy" for the essential hypertension: low sodium, low calorie diet, blind weight limitation and sodium diuretics, sodium substitutes, often creates iatrogenic hypovolemia and iatrogenic MTLP in such patients.
Note: Intrauterine growth retardation (IUGR) and small for gestational age (SGA) fetuses are commonly seen in malnourished women suffering hypovolemia before clinical signs of MTLP in all groups. Knowledge of your patient's nutritional and emotional status and family history aids tremendously in accurate diagnosis and hence in rational, scientific clinical management.

It is also important to make the same sort of differential diagnosis for the two other traditional signs of MTLP, edema or swelling from water retention, and protein in the urine (commonly termed "albuminuria" or "proteinuria").

There are three major categories of clinical edema in human pregnancy:

1. Physiological edema which involves the lower extremities in about 90% of normal pregnancies and involves the fingers, hands, face in 50%. Large babies, twins, triplets, etc. are apt to have more benign edema and earlier in gestation. In the well nourished pregnant woman such increased water retention is often a good diagnostic sign that multiple fetuses are present.

2. Pathological edema associated with malnutrition during pregnancy and MTLP, especially deficiencies of proteins of high biological quality, calories from carbohydrates, salt and associated deficiencies of vitamins and other minerals.

3. Pathological edema associated with other medical and surgical diseases which can occur in the non-pregnant state or in a man: nephritis, nephrosis, congestive heart failure, liver diseases and many others.

Proteinuria is commonly caused by vaginal or cervical secretions contaminating the urine specimen if the mother is not instructed to get a clean-catch, midstream specimen. It is commonly caused by urinary tract infections and other kidney diseases not related to MTLP. Proteinuria associated with MTLP usually occurs after the disease is well-advanced, but severe MTLP has been observed in the absence of proteinuria.

SALT IN PREGNANCY

Closely allied to the question of hypertension in pregnancy is the question of dietary salt, NaCl. Salt has been blindly restricted in the diets of pregnant women, and especially in MTLP, by Western obstetrics for over 150 years. The classic work of Margaret Robinson at St. Thomas Hospital, London, "Salt in Pregnancy," (*Lancet* 1:178, 1958) convinced me that this traditional, blind salt restriction is wrong in human prenatal care. Consequently I had never advised pregnant women in my prenatal care-nutrition education program to "cut back on salt" nor did I ever use a low sodium diet. Robinson had reported twice as many perinatal infant deaths and two and one-half times more cases of "pre-eclamptic toxemia" among one thousand pregnant women told to follow a "low salt diet" compared to a thousand put on a "high salt diet." There were more abnormal placentas in the low salt group.

The work of Ruth Pike et al. at Penn State (*Internatl. J. Gynecol. Obstet.* 10:1, 1972), who produced low birth weight rat pups with dietary salt restriction alone and studied the renin-angiotensin-aldosterone system in normal and salt-depleted pregnant rats, convinced me that salt is an important essential nutrient for all pregnant mammals including human beings. Thus in 1972 I began to stress to my prenatal patients: "Salt to taste!" with the same enthusiasm and insistence that I had been using to promote high biological quality proteins, adequate calories and other essential nutrients found in a "balanced diet." (*Obstet. Gynecol.* 40:868, 1972)

WEIGHT GAIN IN PREGNANCY

Many studies in the last fifteen years have confirmed my position that weight limitation to any "magic numbers" or "pattern of gain" has no scientific basis whatsoever and is in fact harmful to large numbers of pregnant women. (see Annotated Bibliography, Apppendix) If her doctor recommends *any* arbitrary number as an "upper limit" or ceiling, when the pregnant patient approaches this number or reaches it, she is classically warned to "cut down" on her intakes of foods and salt. This advice to starve usually comes during the last half of gestation when the nutritional needs of the pregnant women are increasing daily in the quantitative sense. Thus raising the number of the ceiling begs the question and in no way solves the universal problem of iatrogenic starvation in human prenatal care.

Women with twins gain more weight earlier in gestation than women with a single fetus when they eat to appetite and salt to taste. The total weight gained in a pregnancy with multiple fetuses is more with adequate diets. When the diagnosis of twins is not made prenatally (perhaps in 40% of cases in the USA), blind weight limitation can be disastrous to both mother and babies. MTLP, low birth weight and prematurity have long been associated with twin pregnancy, and the nutritional etiology of this reproductive pathology is now clear. Following the empirical observations of Mrs. Agnes Higgins in the Montreal Diet Dispensary, I advised mothers-to-be with twins to add 30 grams of high quality protein and 500 calories to their diets for each extra fetus; these amounts of protein and calories are present in one quart of milk.

It has been demonstrated beyond all scientific doubt that

normal pregnancy for both mother and baby can occur over a wide range of total weight gain and with many different patterns of gain among adequately nourished women. The late Professor Nicholson J. Eastman of Johns Hopkins University, Dept. of Obstetrics, on June 30, 1968, told a small group of physicians at the NIH in Bethesda, Maryland:

"I taught the wrong ideas about weight gain in pregnancy all my professional life."

He made this statement after presenting some of the preliminary data from the NIH Collaborative Study of Cerebral Palsy and from his own studies of weight gain in pregnancy at Johns Hopkins. (Eastmans, N.J. et al. *Obstet: Gynecol. Surv.* 23:1003, (1968).

SALT DIURETICS IN PREGNANCY

In the fall of 1958 the USA Food and Drug Administration, Bureau of Drugs, approved a potent oral salt diuretic, chlorothiazide (Merck, Sharp & Dohme's DIURIL®), for use in "edema of pregnancy," "toxemia of pregnancy (eclampsia)," and for "hypertension in pregnancy." Eventually ten other major "ethical" drug companies joined in this assault on maternal-fetal health. (see page —— above) Someday this will be recognized as the gravest, most terrible error in modern "legal drug abuse." It became a worldwide problem.

Professor Bo S. Lindberg writing in 1979 on "Salt, diuretics and pregnancy" (*Gynecol. obstet. Invest.* 10:145, 1979) observed that even in Sweden over ten thousand pregnancies each year have been subjected to these diuretic drugs on no scientific basis whatsoever.

Since 1958 I have been involved in a struggle to expose this cruel drug industry fraud, a hoax so extensive, pervasive, and persistent to this day that it staggers the imagination. The fraudulent "research" on which the drug industry based its aggressive "hard sell" of sodium diuretics in human pregnancy was fully exposed at a public hearing of the FDA Bureau of Drugs, OB-GYN Advisory Committee in Rockville, Maryland on July 17, 1975. Professor Leon Chesley of the Dept. OB-GYN, SUNY Downstate Medical Center, Brooklyn, New York, for thirty years one of the nation's leading researchers in this field, reviewed the major "research" papers which the drug industry had used to support their claims for the "efficacy and safety" of thiazide diuretics in human pregnancy. Chesley demonstrated these reports were complete frauds. Not one representative of the drug industry appeared to try to defend the now obvious, often lethal errors of using salt diuretics in malnourished, hypovolemic, hypoproteinemic, toxemic patients.

Almost seven years have passed since that hearing and the FDA still rigidly refuses to *contraindicate* use of sodium diuretics in pregnancy "without more hard data." It is important to remember that there never were any scientific, "hard" data whatsoever which supported the diuretics-in-pregnancy fraud. The widespread, uncritical acceptance and massive use of these drugs in pregnancy occurred because of profound physician ignorance of the basic principles of human maternal-fetal physiology and of applied nutrition science, and also because of the rigid refusal of the medical profession in the United States to recognize the role of malnutrition during pregnancy in causing major reproductive pathology.

PATHOLOGY OF METABOLIC TOXEMIA
OF LATE PREGNANCY

Because MTLP is a primary metabolic-hepatic disease caused by malnutrition during pregnancy, I had tried in 1966 to focus attention on the specific liver pathology long observed to be characteristic of this disease by workers all over the world: periportal hemorrhagic necrosis, infarction and fatty infiltration. It is still my opinion that adequate nutrition and normal liver function throughout gestation prevent these lesions.

In 1973 Sheehan and Lynch of Liverpool published *Pathology of Toxaemia of Pregnancy* (Edinburgh and London: Churchill Livingston), a monumental review of over 1,700 references with their own study of 677 autopsies on obstetric patients; 377 of these women had died with "toxaemia of pregnancy." In toxemic women they described a variety of specific liver lesions which were never observed in women dying in pregnancy from causes not associated with "toxaemia of pregnancy." The kidney lesions found in women dying of "toxaemia of pregnancy" were considered by Sheehan and Lynch of minor significance, not severe enough to cause much impairment of renal function nor to contribute to the cause of maternal death. (see: *World Medical Journal*, vol. 21, p. 70, 1974) Cerebral hemorrhage and infarction were considered to be major causes of maternal deaths.

THOMAS H. BREWER, M.D.
Bedford Hills, N.Y.
May, 1982

A NEW ANNOTATED BIBLIOGRAPHY OF SCIENTIFIC STUDIES

Nutrition in Pregnancy: A New Annotated Bibliography of Scientific Studies

(reprinted with permission of the Society for the Protection of the Unborn through Nutrition, Chicago, copyright 1982)

INTRODUCTION

SPUN publishes this annotated bibliography to help those interested and concerned people who want to explore the unequivocal role of foods, salt, water, and drugs in determining the outcome of human pregnancy. Presented is a representative sample of decades of international research and practical clinical observations which have documented that prenatal malnutrition is the predominant cause of maternal complications and a continuum of neurological, physical, motor, and behavioral abnormalities in the offspring. In fact, SPUN recognizes that maternal nutrition is as vital to maternal/fetal and neonatal health as the regular intake of oxygen.

This concept remains an unpopular point of view in U.S. obstetrics and nutrition science in 1982. The entire field is considered "controversial" by practicing physicians and research academics alike, but pregnant women and their families need correct, scientific, practical knowledge *now*, such as that which we have compiled.

The *protective effects* of enough good foods, salt and water and the dangers of harmful drugs have been demonstrated by researchers and practitioners all over the world, and yet since no "ethical" research worker can starve a pregnant woman under experimental conditions (as animal nutrition scientists are able to do), nutritional nonchalance and neglect continue to characterize the traditional prenatal care which pregnant women still receive in the U.S. in 1982. Contemporary textbooks of obstetrics, perinatology,

[155]

internal medicine, pediatrics and even nutrition science still regard some of the works and point of view in this bibliography as "unscientific" simply because these studies establish a *causal* relationship, not just a statistical association, between malnutrition during pregnancy and major maternal/fetal and neonatal complications. Disregarding this direct cause-and-effect relationship is institutionalized among academicians in obstetrics, nursing, public health, nutrition and other professions who preoccupy themselves with unlimited, meaningless abstractions while neglecting the basic principles of ensuring maternal and newborn *health*.

The irrational, unscientific use of restrictive diets in prenatal care, i.e., low-protein, low-calorie and low-salt diets, has been thoroughly documented as being *harmful* to both the mother and her unborn child. Moreover, the blind use of "weight limitation" in pregnancy management has been exposed by clinical observations on many thousands of pregnancies and has been shown to be dangerous since it leads to malnutrition, especially in the last half of gestation.

This bibliography offers a foundation for sane obstetrical practices *now* which can make *primary prevention* of metabolic toxemia of late pregnancy, abruptio placentae, severe infections, low birth weight and brain damage a reality for all pregnant women and their unborn babies regardless of age, parity, race or socioeconomic status. It is essential that both mother and fetus be protected from all harmful drugs, other dangerous chemicals, and radiation as well as from the obvious ravages of prenatal malnutrition.

I. CLINICAL OBSERVATIONS AND RESEARCH

1. Ross, Robert A. "Relation of vitamin deficiency to the toxemia of pregnancy." *So. Med. J.* 28:120, 1935.

    In North Carolina, he identified the role of malnutrition and poverty in eclampsia and other human reproductive casualty.

2. Strauss, M. B. "Observations on the etiology of the toxemias of pregnancy." *Am. J. Med. Sci.* 190:811, 1935.

    Internist at Harvard recognized the role of protein and

related deficiencies in the etology of eclampsia. Toxemia subsided in women placed on a 260-gram protein, well-balanced diet with injections of vitamin B.

3. DODGE, E., and FROST, T. "Relation between blood plasma proteins and toxemias of pregnancy." *JAMA* 111:1398, 1938.

The authors observed that low-protein diets, often prescribed by physicians for the treatment of toxemia of pregnancy, increased the severity of the disease. They successfully improved the condition with diets consisting of six or more eggs daily, one to two quarts of milk, lean meat, legumes and other nutritious foods; and they directly linked toxemia with low serum albumin and inadequate protein intake.

4. TOMPKINS, WINSLOW T. "The significance of nutritional deficiency in pregnancy: A preliminary report." *J. Intl. Col. Surg.* 4:147, 1941.

Eradicated preeclampsia/eclampsia, low birth weight, and stillbirth at Philadelphia Lying-in Hospital. Infant mortality was reduced to 4 per 1,000 births.

5. BURKE, BERTHA S., et al. "Nutrition studies during pregnancy." *Am. J. Obstet. Gynecol.* 46:38, 1943.

Confirmed nutritional thesis of the etiology of eclampsia and demonstrated the protective effects of adequate nutrition on the mother, fetus/neonate and infant.

6. CAMERON, C. S., and GRAHAM, S. "Antenatal diet and its influence on stillbirths and prematurity." *Glasgow Med. J.* 24:1, 1944.

In both prospective and retrospective studies, maternal malnutrition was found to cause low birth weight, stillbirth, and infant mortality.

7. ANTONOV, A. N. "Children born during the siege of Leningrad in 1942." *J. Pediatrics* 30:250, 1947.

War-caused famine led to widespread infertility, amenorrhea, a low-birth-weight incidence of 49%, and infant mortality of 500 per 1,000 live births.

8. MITCHELL, J., et al. "Dietary habits of a group of severe preeclamptics in Alabama." *J. Natl. Med. Assn.* 41:122, 1949.

Toxemia was found to be closely associated with inadequate nutrition. When placed on a sound diet providing, on the average, 124 grams of protein per day, all of the toxemic women improved.

9. FERGUSON, JAMES H. "Maternal death in the rural South: A study of forty-seven consecutive cases." *JAMA* 146:1388, 1951.

   The author described the severe poverty and malnutrition of toxemic women in rural Mississippi.

10. HAMLIN, REGINALD. "The prevention of eclampsia and preeclampsia." *Lancet* 1:64, 1952.

    Eradicated eclampsia by an aggressive nutrition education program in a public prenatal clinic, Women's Hospital, Sydney, Australia.

11. TOMPKINS, W., and WIEHL, D. "Nutrition and nutritional deficiencies as related to the premature." *Pediatric Clin. No. Am.* 1:687, 1954.

    Weight at birth was highly associated with prenatal nutrition, weight gain during pregnancy, and prepregnancy weight. The low-birth-weight incidence among women who received protein and vitamin supplementation, gained substantial weight during pregnancy, and were not underweight at conception was less than 2%. In contrast, 24% of the babies born to women most likely to be malnourished were underweight at birth.

12. KNOBLOCH, H., et al. "Neuropsychiatric sequelae of prematurity: A longitudinal study." *JAMA* 161:581, 1956.

    A well-controlled and meticulously designed longitudinal scientific study linking low birth weight to neurological dysfunction and impaired cognitive potential.

13. ROBINSON, MARGARET. "Salt in pregnancy." *Lancet* 1:178, 1958.

    Classic study at St. Thomas Hospital, London. Among 2,000 pregnant women, those put on a "low-sodium diet" experimentally had over twice the incidence of toxemia and significantly higher perinatal mortality than those told to "eat more salt." This study should not have been done because it was unphysiological and needlessly harmed many mothers and babies.

14. BREWER, T. H. "Limitations of diuretic therapy in the management of severe toxemia: The significance of hypoalbuminemia." *Am. J. Obstet. Gynecol.* 83:1352, 1962.

    First published account of the threat diuretics pose to the health of mothers and their unborns by attacking maternal and fetal plasma volumes. This warning went unheeded, as the use of sodium diuretics became a routine practice in prenatal care among most obstetricians in the U.S.

15. GREEN, G. H. "Maternal mortality in the toxaemias of pregnancy." *Aus. N.Z. J. Obstet. Gynaecol.* 2:145, 1962.

Ten toxemic women died in hypovolemic shock, without excess blood loss or infection.

16. BREWER, T. H. "Administration of human serum albumin in severe acute toxaemia of pregnancy." *J. Obstet. Gynaecol. Br. Cwlth.* 70:1001, 1963.

Rejected by editors of U.S. medical journals, this paper demonstrated the nutritional pathogenesis of metabolic toxemia of late pregnancy, stressing the problem of maternal hypovolemia.

17. BREWER, T. H. "Human pregnancy nutrition: A clinical view." *Obstet. Gynecol.* 30:605, 1967.

Advocates application of scientific nutrition and physiology in human prenatal care.

18. IYENGAR, LEELA. "Urinary estrogen excretion in undernourished pregnant Indian women: Effect of dietary supplement on urinary estrogens and birth weights of infants." *Am. J. Obstet. Gynecol.* 102:834, 1968.

Demonstrated beneficial effects on fetal growth by improving maternal diets as late as the 36th week of gestation.

19. BREWER, T. H. "A case of recurrent abruptio placentae." *Del. Med. J.* 41:325, 1969.

Dietary history recorded of a woman who had two abruptions and two neonatal deaths of low-birth-weight babies in one year. After her malnutrition was corrected, she had a normal baby with no complications.

20. BLETKA, M., et al. "Volume of whole blood and absolute amount of serum proteins in the early stage of late toxemia of pregnancy." *Am. J. Obstet. Gynecol.* 106:10, 1970.

Valuable observation documenting that hypovolemia and hypoalbuminemia precede hypertension and other signs of metabolic toxemia of late pregnancy.

21. BREWER, T. H: "Human pregnancy nutrition: An examination of traditional assumptions." *Aus. N.Z.J. Obstet. Gynaecol.* 10:87, 1970.

Exposes the incorrect ideology and dangers of the routine obstetrical practices of weight control, salt restriction and the use of sodium diuretics.

22. DUFFUS, G. M., et al. "The relationship between baby weight and changes in maternal weight, total body water, plasma volume, electrolytes and proteins and urinary oestriol excretion." *J. Obstet. Gynaecol. Br. Cwlth.* 78:97, 1971.

Total circulating protein mass correlated most significantly with infant birth weight.

23. PLATT, B. S., and STEWART, R. J. C. "Reversible and irreversible effects of protein-calorie deficiency on the central nervous system of animals and man." *World Rev. Nutr. Diet.* 13:43, 1971.

Neurological dysfunction is extensively linked to malnutrition in both animal and human studies in this review of 177 works.

24. BREWER, T. H. "Human maternal-fetal nutrition." *Obstet. Gynecol.* 40:868, 1972.

Another call for the application of physiology and basic nutrition science in human prenatal care. This paper criticizes the position of the American College of Obstetricians and Gynecologists in this field; i.e., "Nothing is known."

25. HIBBARD, LESTER. "Maternal mortality due to acute toxemia." *Obstet. Gynecol.* 42:263, 1973.

Reports alarming increase in maternal deaths from metabolic toxemia of late pregnancy. Most of the toxemic women had been placed on low-salt and/or low-calorie diets. Some were also given sodium diuretics.

26. BREWER, T. H. "Metabolic toxemia of late pregnancy in a county prenatal nutrition education project: A preliminary report." *J. Reprod. Med.* 13:175, 1974.

Data from National Institutes of Health retrospective study of 5,615 pregnancies delivered in Contra Costa County, California, 1965-70, a 5½-year period. No cases of eclampsia were found, nor was there any maternal death in the nutrition project pregnancies. Not one woman had a Cesarean for "severe preeclampsia" or "hypertension."

27. GRIEVE, J. F. K. "Prevention of gestational failure by high protein diet." *J. Reprod. Med.* 13:170, 1974.

Through nutrition education in his prenatal clinics and by hospitalizing malnourished pregnant women for nutritional therapy, viz., "a pound of red meat every day," an OB/GYN physician in Motherwell, Scotland, eradicated eclampsia and abruptio placentae. The incidence of perinatal death was reduced more than twentyfold.

28. HABICHT, J. P., et al. "Relation of maternal supplementary feeding during pregnancy to birth weight and other sociobiological factors," in *Nutrition and Fetal Development*. M. Winick, ed. New York: John Wiley & Sons, 1974.

Caloric supplementation among low-income women resulted in eradication of stillbirth and a reduction of the incidence of low birth weight from 13.4% to 3.5%. Demonstrates the protein-sparing effects of calories from carbohydrates and fats among women on low-protein diets.

29. HOWARD, PEGGY. "Albumin concentrate can be used for preeclampsia." *OB/GYN News*, October 1, 1974.

All of the toxemic women given 50 grams of serum albumin daily gave birth to babies in good health. Infusions of serum albumin improved renal function, increased estriol excretion, prevented eclamptic convulsions, and resulted in a reduction in perinatal mortality to onefourth the rate of the "controls" and eradication of abruptio placentae.

30. BREWER, T. H. "Consequences of malnutrition in human pregnancy." *CIBA Review: Perinatal Medicine*, pp. 5-6. Basel, Switzerland: CIBA-Geigy, Ltd., 1975.

Discusses the role of malnutrition, including iatrogenic malnutrition, via physician-prescribed low-calorie, low-sodium diets and sodium diuretics in the etiology of metabolic toxemia of late pregnancy, abruptio placentae, low birth weight, prematurity, severe infections and brain damage in children. Another call for applied science in this field on the clinical level in human prenatal care.

31. LECHTIG, A., et al. "Effect of moderate maternal malnutrition on the placenta." *Am. J. Obstet. Gynecol.* 123:191, 1975.

Placental weight, associated with birth weight, increased with caloric supplementation, providing more evidence of the protein-sparing effect of calories.

32. HIGGINS, AGNES C. "Nutritional status and the outcome of pregnancy." *J. Can. Diet. Assn.* 37:17, 1976.

Documents the value of nutrition education and food supplementation in increasing birth weight, lowering infant mortality, and eradicating eclampsia.

33. MATTHEWS, D. D., et al. "Modern trends in management of non-albuminuric hypertension in late pregnancy." *Br. Med. J.* 2:623, 1978.

Challenges the traditional therapies of hypertension in pregnancy: bed rest, sedation, low-sodium diets and sodium diuretics and pre-term induction. These are shown to be of no value or harmful. The authors still exhibit no conception of the role of malnutrition in causing hypovolemia.

34. PORAPAKKHAM, SAROJ. "An epidemiological study of eclampsia." *Obstet. Gynecol.* 54:26, 1979.

Reports on 298 cases of eclampsia involving 14 maternal deaths in one hospital in Bangkok, Thailand, among malnourished women, many of whom were given furosemide.

35. LAURENCE, K. M., et al. "Increased risk of recurrence of pregnancies complicated by fetal neural tube defects in mothers receiving poor diets, and possible benefit of dietary counseling." *Br. Med. J.* 281:1592, 1980.

Prospective and retrospective studies indicated that the second most common birth defect in the U.S. is preventable by sound nutrition. The incidence of neural tube defects was 18% in a control group of poorly nourished mothers.

II. BOOKS, REVIEWS, AND ACADEMIC, STATISTICAL AND EPIDEMIOLOGICAL STUDIES

1. ACOSTA-SISON, HONORA. "Relation between state of nutrition of the mother and the birth weight of the fetus: A preliminary study." *J. Philippine Islands Med. Assn.* 9:174, 1929.

The incidence of low birth weight was found to be nearly ten times higher among poorly nourished women than in those determined to have good nutritional status.

2. MELLANBY, EDWARD. "Nutrition and child-bearing." *Lancet* 2:1131, 1933.

Discussed the need for protective nutrients in human pregnancy and theorized that eclampsia is a metabolic, nutrition-deficiency disease. He noted: "Nutrition is the most important of all environmental factors in childbearing whether the problem be considered from the point of view of the mother or that of the offspring."

3. THEOBALD, G. W. "Discussion on diet in pregnancy." *Proc. R. Soc. Med.* 28:1388, 1935.

Refuting various speculations about the causes of toxemia, the author concluded that its etiology is malnutrition.

4. EBBS, JOHN, et al. "The influence of prenatal diet on the mother and child." *J. Nutr.* 22:515, 1941.

The low-birth-weight incidence was 2.2% in the best nourished group.

5. BALFOUR, M. I. "Nutrition of expectant and nursing mothers. Interim report of the People's League for Health." *Lancet* 2:10, 1942.

Food supplementation and nutrition education contributed to significant reductions in toxemia, perinatal death and maternal mortality.

6. ROSS, ROBERT A. "Late toxemias of pregnancy: The number one obstetrical problem of the South." *Am. J. Obstet. Gynecol.* 54:723, 1947.

This grim report showed that the toxemia incidence and infant mortality were high among the malnourished poor.

7. TOVERUD, GUTTORM. "The influence of nutrition on the course of pregnancy." *Milbank Mem. Fund Qtr.* 28:7, 1950.

Proper nutrition reduced the incidence of low birth weight to 2.2% and halved that of stillbirths.

8. JEANS, P. C., et al. "Incidence of prematurity in relation to maternal nutrition." *J. Am. Diet. Assn.* 31:576, 1955.

Low birth weight was found to be highly correlated to prenatal malnutrition.

9. KNOBLOCH, H., and PASAMANICK, B. "Prospective studies on the epidemiology of reproductive casualty: Methods, findings, and some implications." *Merrill-Palmer Qtr. Behav. Dev.* 12:27, 1966.

Maternal health is linked directly to child development.

10. PASAMANICK, B., and KNOBLOCH, H. "Retrospective studies on the epidemiology of reproductive casualty: Old and new." *Merrill-Palmer Qtr. Behav. Dev.* 12:7, 1966.

A continuum of neuropsychiatric disorders in this review of 49 scientific studies is associated with low birth weight and the presence of complications during pregnancy.

11. SCHNEIDER, JAN. "Low birth weight infants." *Obstet. Gynecol.* 31:283, 1968.

    Documents the alarming rise in low birth weight in the U.S. after 1950.

12. SINGER, J. E., et al. "Relationship of weight gain during pregnancy to birth weight and infant growth and development in the first year of life." *Obstet. Gynecol.* 31:417, 1968.

    Weight gain during pregnancy is statistically related to birth weight and infant mental, neurological, and motor function. Unfortunately, the paper ignores the question of the quality of diet causing the weight gain.

13. DRILLIEN, C. M. "School disposal and performance for children of different birthweight born 1953-1960." *Arch. Dis. Child.* 44:562, 1969.

    Low birth weight is associated with an increased proneness to handicaps and a lowered I.Q. Birth weight was found to influence a child's development more than socioeconomic background.

14. WINICK, M., and ROSSO, P. "The effect of severe early malnutrition on cellular growth of human brain." *Pediatric Res.* 3:181, 1969.

    Malnutrition during pregnancy is shown to lead to a significant reduction of brain cells in the newborn. Impaired hyperplasia of brain cells was reflected in their finding that brain weight, protein, RNA and DNA were substantially reduced in newborns of malnourished women.

15. PIKE, R. L., and GURSKY, D. S. "Further evidence of deleterious effects produced by sodium restriction during pregnancy." *Am. J. Clin. Nutr.* 23:883, 1970.

    The consequences of sodium deficiency, such as hypovolemia and stress on the renin-angiotensin-aldosterone homeostasis, are well documented.

16. BREWER, T. H. "Disease and Social Class," in *The Social Responsibility of the Scientist*. Martin Brown, ed. New York: Free Press, 1971.

    Examines mechanisms by which poverty and malnutrition cause human diseases, including maternal and infant morbidity and mortality. Stresses the need for *primary prevention*.

17. FORT, A. T. "Adequate prenatal nutrition." *Obstet. Gynecol.*

37:286, 1971.

Proper fetal development and birth weight, the author states, are directly dependent upon the pregnant woman's nutritional intake.

18. SCHEWITZ, L. "Hypertension and renal disease in pregnancy." *Med. Clin. No. Am.* 55:47, 1971.

This erudite review of 100 studies demonstrated the absence of scientific validity in prescribing a low-salt diet and/or sodium diuretics to edematous or hypertensive expectant mothers. Severely hypertensive pregnant women received 14 grams of salt daily without demonstrable harmful effects or increased blood pressures.

19. CHESLEY, LEON C. "Plasma volume and red cell volume in pregnancy." *Am. J. Obstet. Gynecol.* 112:440, 1972.

Leading expert in the field of "preeclampsia/eclampsia" condemns the use of sodium diuretics in toxemic patients because of their hypovolemic state. Subsequently, his highly regarded chapter entitled "The Hypertensive Diseases of Pregnancy" was dropped from Dr. Jack Pritchard's edition of *Williams Obstetrics*.

20. KELMAN, L., et al. "Effects of dietary protein restriction on albumin synthesis, albumin catabolism, and the plasma aminogram." *Am. J. Clin. Nutr.* 25:1174, 1972.

A valuable study done on men in South Africa which demonstrates the critical role of dietary protein intake in maintaining hepatic synthesis of serum albumin. Such studies in which daily protein intakes were reduced to 10 grams cannot be done ethically on human pregnancies, they demonstrate the pernicious effects of both low-protein and low-calorie diets.

21. LOWE, C. U. "Research in infant nutrition: The untapped well." *Am. J. Clin. Nutr.* 25:245, 1972.

Emphasizes that the abandonment of weight control, low-salt diets, and diuretics is necessary to significantly reduce the rates of prematurity and low birth weight.

22. PIKE, RUTH L., and SMICIKLAS, H. "A reappraisal of sodium restriction during pregnancy." *Intl. J. Gynaecol. Obstet.* 10:1, 1972.

Demonstrates that salt is an essential, protective nutrient for human pregnancy and not a "poison," as is still believed by many OB/GYN physicians in the U.S.

23. FOOTE, R. G., et al. "The use of liberal salt diet in preeclamptic toxaemia and essential hypertension with pregnancy." *New Zealand Med. J.* 77:242, 1973.

   More clinical observations which destroy the "salt is a killer" myth in human pregnancy.

24. BREWER, T. H. "Iatrogenic starvation in human pregnancy." *Medikon* 4:14, 1974.

   A call for major changes in current U.S. OB/GYN nutrition and drug practices in antenatal care. Advocates that constructive actions be taken immediately to improve human maternal/fetal and neonatal health in the U.S. and to protect all pregnant women and their unborns from the ravages of prenatal malnutrition and harmful drugs.

25. BREWER, T. H. "Pancreatitis in pregnancy." *J. Reprod. Med.* 12:204, 1974.

   Another painful, often fatal complication of pregnancy linked to the use of sodium diuretics and low-sodium, low-calorie diets.

26. BREWER, T. H. "Toxemia—A disease of prejudice?" *World Med. J.* 21:70, 1974.

   Includes a review of *Pathology of Toxaemia of Pregnancy* by H. L. Sheehan and J. B. Lynch (Edinburgh and London: Churchill Livingstone, 1973). A great deal of emphasis is placed on the specific liver pathology associated with eclampsia.

27. SHNEOUR, E. *The Malnourished Mind.* New York: Doubleday, 1974.

   Discusses, in a conversational manner, the unequivocal causal relationship between impaired development and malnutrition during pregnancy, infancy and childhood. Refutes the myth that mental deficiency is largely caused by genetic factors.

28. WILLIAMS, PHYLLIS S. *Nourishing Your Unborn Child.* New York: Avon, 1974.

   A useful guide for pregnant women, containing valuable information on pregnancy physiology, the role and sources of various nutrients, and 163 pages of menus and recipes.

29. BREWER, T. H. "Etiology of eclampsia." *Am. J. Obstet. Gynecol.* 127:448, 1977.

   Refutes the age-old myth that eclampsia is a disease limited to the first pregnancy and another myth that it is caused by an occult "utero-placental ischemia." The well-nourished primigravida, protected from hypovolemia (the real cause of "utero-placental ischemia") all through gestation, *never develops eclampsia.*

30. BREWER, T. H., and HODIN, JAY. "Why Women Must Meet the Nutritional Stress of Pregnancy," in *21st Century Obstetrics Now!* Stewart and Stewart, ed. Marble Hill, Mo.: NAPSAC Press, 1977.

   Cites 143 references linking maternal malnutrition to a continuum of perinatal complications.

31. WILLIAMS, SUE RODWELL. "Nutrition During Pregnancy and Lactation," in *Nutrition and Diet Therapy,* 3d ed. St. Louis: C. V. Mosby Co., 1977.

   An excellent textbook providing a wealth of information about basic nutrition science and its application on the clinical level. The first nutrition textbook to break with the traditional "nothing is known" position regarding the role of prenatal malnutrition in causing human reproductive casualty, including metabolic toxemia of late pregnancy.

32. BREWER, T. H. "The 'No-Risk' Pregnancy Diet," in *The Pregnancy After 30 Workbook.* Gail Sforza Brewer, ed. Emmaus, Pa.: Rodale Press, 1978.

   Provides the expectant mother with the guidance she needs to maintain good health and give birth to a healthy, fully developed child. Valuable for women of any age.

33. *Preventing Nutritional Complications of Pregnancy: A Manual for SPUN Counselors.* Chicago: SPUN, 1978.

   A practical reference for those who wish to teach applied scientific nutrition and physiology to pregnant women. Concludes with a practical quiz of 25 questions.

34. BREWER, GAIL SFORZA. *What Every Pregnant Woman Should Know: The Truth About Diets and Drugs in Pregnancy.* New York: Penguin, 1979.

   An extremely valuable guide for the expectant mother. The author discusses physiological adjustments of pregnancy and how to meet its nutritional stresses. To help the expectant mother maintain proper nutritional status, 92 pages of menus and recipes are included. Of equal importance to the reader is the book's discussion of the history of all aspects of the Thalidomide II regimen (low-calorie and/or low-salt diets, blind weight limitations, use of sodium diuretics and amphetamines, etc.) to provide her with the confidence she needs to reject any regimen of nutritional mismanagement imposed by her health professionals.

35. SHANKLIN, DOUGLAS, and HODIN, JAY. *Maternal Nutrition and Child Health*. Springfield, Ill.: C. C. Thomas, 1979.

 This book, highly recommended for the health care professional and others desiring scientific documentation of the role of malnutrition in human reproductive casualty, is a near-exhaustive review of prospective and retrospective scientific studies, physiological and neurological evidence, and epidemiological reviews linking prenatal malnutrition to a wide spectrum of perinatal complications. Containing 77 tables and graphs, the work cites 239 references. This book is an excellent antidote for the contemporary institutionalized nonchalance in the field of applied preventive nutrition prevalent among health care professionals.

36. BREWER, GAIL SFORZA. *Lo Que Toda Mujer Embarazada Debe Saber: La Verdad Acerca de las Dietas y las Medicinas Durante el Embarazo*. Mexico, D.F.: Editorial Diana, S.A., 1980.

 Spanish translation of number 34.

37. GORMICAN, ANNETTE, et al. "Relationships of maternal weight gain, prepregnancy weight and infant birthweight." *J. Am. Diet. Assn.* 77:662, 1980.

 A retrospective controlled study documented that weight control and salt restriction significantly reduced birth weight and resulted in other deleterious consequences.

38. NOBLE, ELIZABETH. *Having Twins*. Boston: Houghton Mifflin, 1980.

 An absolutely unique book in that it recognizes and deals with the increased nutritional stresses of multiple fetuses and presents SPUN's ideology and practical diet adapted for multiple births.

39. "Prenatal nutritional counseling substantially reduces low birth weight deliveries." *Group Health News*, March 1980.

 A voluntary prenatal nutrition education program at a Health Maintenance Organization resulted in a 61% reduction in the incidence of underweight births in addition to a significant decline in infant morbidity and mortality.

40. BREWER, GAIL, and GREENE, JANICE. *Right from the Start.* Emmaus, Pa.: Rodale Press, 1981.

Incorporates the nutritional perspective on all aspects of fetal development, labor and delivery, breastfeeding, and the first month after birth for mother and baby.

41. KENEFICK, MADELEINE. *Positively Pregnant.* Los Angeles. Pinnacle Books, 1981.

Containing a foreword by SPUN's President, Tom Brewer, M.D., the book appropriately proceeds to recommend SPUN's diet, outline the specific role of nutrition in contributing to maternal health and fetal development, maintain an emphatic position against the use of physician-imposed restrictive diets and drugs, and discuss effective, commonsense approaches in treating pregnancy-related complications. In contrast to other books which imply that pregnancy is a pathological process or, at best, fail to convey its pleasant aspects, the author successfully incorporated a balance of factual, practical information with humor while interspersing her personal experiences during pregnancy. Pregnant women, who will also benefit from the book's 148 reference citations, useful glossary, and several illustrations, will find it delightful reading.

III. THE SOCIETY FOR THE PROTECTION OF THE UNBORN THROUGH NUTRITION (SPUN)

SPUN was founded in 1972 in Chicago as a not-for-profit, educational, tax exempt corporation to help improve human maternal-fetal health in the United States by every legal means possible.

Through the organization's multitude of educational services —which include the publication and distribution of materials for both pregnant women and health care professionals; involvement at training seminars for obstetrics practitioners and childbirth educators; presentations at workshops and conferences; prenatal nutrition counseling; referrals; and a hotline service— tens of thousands of individuals have become enlightened on the most effective means of safeguarding maternal and infant health. Due largely to its efforts, trends have been established for physicians becoming more nutrition conscious and, therefore, tolerating increased weight gains, recommending that the pregnant woman salt her food to taste, and abandoning the use of diuretics. In fact, SPUN played an active role in the initiation of and participation at an FDA OB/GYN Advisory Committee hearing on the use of diuretics in pregnancy. At the July 17, 1975, hearing, diuretics and low-salt diets were determined to be contraindicated in pregnancy and potentially hazardous, especially in the presence of MTLP. Currently, the organization is involved in a similar campaign to encourage the FDA to withdraw its approval of ritodrine, a drug used to prevent or postpone premature labor, which is more effectively averted by improved nutrition and the abandonment of Thalidomide II practices.

SPUN also provides medical research and recommends expert witnesses when individuals file claims for damage resulting from medical/nutritional mismanagement. In one such case that was decided on September 17, 1977, the organization was instrumental in convincing a jury that the use of a low-calorie/low-protein diet, salt restriction and diuretics caused a child's retardation, thereby establishing for the first time judicial recognition of the consequences of malnutrition during pregnancy.

Membership in SPUN is available to those who are supportive of the organization's educational activities. For an annual fee of $15, members receive a subscription to *The Pregnant Issue*, discounts for materials ordered, and other services.

Mailing address: SPUN
17 N. Wabash, Suite #603
Chicago, IL 60602
SPUN Nutrition/Toxemia/Intervention Hotline: 914-666-5199

IV. METABOLIC TOXEMIA OF LATE PREGNANCY IN THE THIRD WORLD

As U.S. Americans we have a fundamental responsibility to our own people in this field, but we also recognize the worldwide nature of the role of malnutrition during pregnancy in a vast spectrum of preventable human suffering and diseases and deaths of women and babies. That this role can be so distorted, repressed, denied, ignored is one of the modern enigmas of obstetrics in the 1980s. We have received personal communications from physicians who live in Mexico and other Latin American nations, in South Africa and other African nations, in India, in Thailand, in Iran, in Iraq, in Egypt, etc. all of whom have observed a high incidence of MTLP among women in poverty in those nations. Wherever the Western low calorie, low salt diets for blind weight control and use of salt diuretics become popular, MTLP appears with increasing frequency among the upper classes, a result of iatrogenic maternal malnutrition and hypovolemia.

Here are a few recent references from the literature:

AFRICA   *Lancet* 1:146, 1978, Jan. 21
THAILAND   *Obstet. Gynecol.* 54:26, 1979
INDIA   *Am. J. Clin. Nutri.* 34:775, 1981
MEXICO   *Am. J. Obstet. Gynecol.* 142:28, 1982, Jan. 1